BEYOND THE EYE OF THE STORM

A Community Nurse's Tales of Post-Pandemic Perseverance

GEORGE HORNER

To my family and friends for putting up with me writing yet another book. Thanks for the support and I love you all.

Copyright © 2024 by George Horner.

The right of George Horner to be identified as the author of this work has been asserted by him in accordance with the Copyright, Designs and Patents Act 1988.

All rights reserved. No part of this book may be reproduced in any form or by any means – electronic, mechanical, photocopy, recording, scanning, information storage and retrieval systems, without permission in writing from the author. The only exception is by using brief quotations and short excerpts for a review or article, which does not require the written permission of the author.

ISBN: 978-1-7395704-5-3

Cover designed by Sabeeh ul Hassan
Book formatted by Sophie Hanks

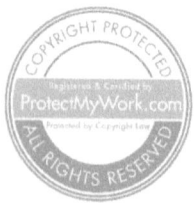

A SECTION ON LEGALITIES:

Last time I wrote a memoir about my personal experiences as a nurse, I was concerned about the legalities of self-publishing my work. I didn't know whether I had done enough to avoid litigation and a breach of my professional contract through my writing. I contacted the Head of Executive Affairs and Projects in my Trust within the National Health Service (NHS), which I also did with this new memoir. I was pleased I did this because I received the support I needed before the publication of my work. I anonymised all staff and colleagues that were mentioned as well as various other personal details. Just like my workings as a healthcare professional, I treated every individual with respect in my writing. Following these steps has allowed my work to be safe for publication and avoiding any characters from being recognisable to anybody. I didn't want some angry niece coming up to me in the middle of the street saying, "Why were you talking about my aunty in your new book? We didn't give you permission to do that?!"

Unlike Hidden Heroes of our Community where I wrote in depth about the national and international news stories during the months of the pandemic, I only dabbled in this now and again in the new book when I felt it was impactful towards my career and personal life. Whenever I did this, I again used trustworthy sources, such as BBC News, The Daily Mail & Telegraph, and literature belonging to the Royal College of Nursing (RCN) and the British Journal of Nursing (BJN). These stories have been written in my own words with my own running commentary to prevent copyright infringement. I've also quoted celebrities, ground-breaking philosophers and politicians and important figures in nursing to influence what I'm writing about, and I believe this to be fair use with no need to seek permission.

The events of this book document my time as a community staff nurse from the start of 2021 to the end of 2023. To respect the privacy of the patients I cared for and the staff I've worked with who may not wish to be recognised, I've anonymised their names and changed other personal information to maintain confidentiality. Some content has been created in stories for dramatic purposes but still relate to other previous clinical cases.

CONTENTS

Introduction - So Why Nursing? 1
1. A New Year with COVID Still Lurking 11
2. One Final Breath 23
3. A Disconnected Family 33
4. Extra Pennies on the Road 39
5. A Challenging Life with Chronic Leg Oedema 47
6. It's Not Just a Sore Foot 59
7. The Complexities of Physical and
   Mental Health Issues 75
8. Every Service Has Its Faults 89
9. Time to Take a Stand 99
10. Away from the Shadows 107
11. An End to a National Treasure 113
12. The Demand for Better Pay 121
13. The Importance of Patient Centred Care 129
14. The Unexpected Appointment 137
15. The Cruelty of a Life-limiting Condition 145

16. A Word of Warning	157
17. Working in Partnership with Residential Homes	169
18. Reporting about the Pressures	177
19. The Importance of Assessing Pain	183
20. When an Incident Becomes Serious	195
21. Opportunity to Self-reflect	203
22. Anticipating a Tragedy	209
23. The Fire Risk	215
24. One Man and His Dog	225
25. A Lone Working Nightmare	231
26. The Festive Patient	243
27. That's a Wrap	251
Acknowledgements	261
Author bio	267

INTRODUCTION
SO WHY NURSING?

Everyone has dreams and aspirations in life. To be successful in some kind of way and achieve life goals. This could be learning a new language or finishing a marathon or running your very own business. Life goals that your childhood self would never have imagined. How about shaking hands with the chancellor on stage at your graduation ceremony after completing a degree not once but twice and then develop in a career you're passionate about. It's only when I look back to my early years at school that I appreciate how much of a positive development journey I took at that time. An example that can be passed down to the next generations, that a strong work ethic goes a hell of a long way. Most of my successes to date are a testament to the solid upbringing my parents provided for me and my two older brothers, keeping us on 'the straight and narrow.' Never pushing us to be the best in whatever we did or telling us who to be, but subtly expecting us to do well in whatever we chose to do. It would only be when we did something naughty or wrong that they'd tell us and show disappointment, and that would be enough to ignite my spark again.

At primary school, I was one of the last in my class to be trusted to use a pen to do any form of writing without the help of a rubber to rectify any spelling mistakes. When it came to secondary school, I started in the lower academic sets in years seven, eight and nine and often had homework sent back with corrections in the teacher's bold, red biro ink, requesting me to redo tasks based on their comments.

I loved my sport, though, and I was classed as one of the top students in football, the track and field events on sports day and field hockey. No matter how lesser the development of my learning was in other subjects, compared with those pupils in the higher sets, I still turned up every school day, hardly having a sick day off, and did my very best in every lesson (bar the occasional distractions from my immature chums and the girls I crushed on).

Even back then, I learnt a valuable lesson that hard work pays dividends. I comprehended this from sporadic projects and assessments, which required a lot of determination. And at times when I turned a corner in my learning, I was awarded a blue A4 piece of card, known as a commendation. It was a way of congratulating me for a decent piece of work, acknowledged by the subject teacher and signed by the headteacher. I was fortunate

So Why Nursing?

to be awarded a few of these at secondary school. When it came to the end of year Prize Giving ceremony at the same school, I was delighted to be summoned to the front of the assembly to shake hands with the headteacher once again and be awarded a book of my choosing that had a small certificate glued to the inner side of the front cover, signifying my accolade. A couple of these books were awarded simply for effort, and you'll find the certificates enclosed in the copies of *Holes* by Louis Sachar and *Harry Potter and the Philosopher's Stone* by J. K Rowling, sitting on my bedroom bookshelf. Alongside them are *Robinson Crusoe* by Daniel Defoe and *Lord of the Flies* by William Golding, awarded as a combination of Effort and Sporting Achievement. If I say so myself, my book taste was damn good back then.

I reaped the rewards of perseverance and commitment at secondary school and bumped up to the higher sets in English and Maths, taking on the more challenging exam papers for my GCSEs in year 11. I was chuffed to bits with the outcome of my results.

During all this time in my education, there wasn't anything promoting the nursing profession. No books, flyers on the walls or speakers in assemblies. I'd see nurses floating around and talking with doctors on TV series like *Holby City* and *Casualty* and in real life when I visited the hospital ward to see a poorly friend or family member. Still, they were a bit alien to me. Nursing seemed like an unknown, unrelatable world in the mind of my younger self. And being a boy, I was surrounded by many other interests and ambitions, which promoted more overt masculinity. I could be a firefighter, a police officer, a mechanic, a welder, an electrician or an engineer. The general personality of these job titles differs from a nurse's gentle, caring approach.

There seemed to be a type of label for male nurses. Stereotyped as being gay in the past, this categorising was still prominent in the nineties and early 00s. In programmes where there's a male nurse, most of the time they'd be a homosexual character. During all that time, I watched American professional wrestling with the characters portraying quite the reverse and often entering the wrestling ring with arm around women in provocative outfits. I was fascinated by the aggression and machismo of these professional athletes, such as Mick Foley, The Undertaker and Dwane Johnson, AKA The Rock from the WWE. My brothers and I would also be inspired by the programme *Gladiators* and would imitate the duelling event from that show by trying to knock each other off the settee with draft excluders. These athletes we watched were a world away from the type of people who work in the profession I pledge my kindness to now.

Moving ahead in my imaginary time-travel machine to my 20s, I had a mischievous side, and in my free time, I acted like one of the lads saying "yes" to every opportunity for house parties and getting wasted at clubs and bars. I look back in disbelief at the numerous occasions when I didn't know my limits with alcohol and when things were taken too far to the point that I'd pass out in places other than somewhere inside my home. My uni days weren't exempt from this either, particularly during my undergraduate degree. The places I can recall include a thorn bush beside the pavement leading to the university campus after a heavy night at the student union bar, shamefully and uncomfortably taking out thorns from both arms the next day in my halls of residence. Another time when I snapped back into reality from an intoxicated state was when I woke up on a farmyard in the early morning after losing my sense of direction to a house I had just started renting when I was studying in Chichester. I was still befuddled as I stood up, stumbling around. Then I had the bright idea of waking the farmer by throwing a stone at his bedroom window to try and ask for a kip on their couch. I then pegged it when I saw his air rifle pointing at me out the window with the warning he'd fire it if I continued trespassing on his property. I later came to my senses with the idea of using Google Maps and remembering what address I lived at.

I never let my drunken antics falter my progress in higher education, though. Once social shenanigans were done and time was needed for essay writing, presentation rehearsing and exam prepping, I directed most of my attention to studying in my bedroom or a quiet library space and knuckled down. I lived a dangerous balance of a 'work hard/play hard' lifestyle, and I came out the other side with a qualification grade I was proud of. My mentality was the same in my postgraduate degree in Adult Nursing.

In between my undergraduate sports degree and my postgraduate nursing degree, I started my first full-time minimum-wage job supporting the learning of children and young adults with physical and learning disabilities. It was at that point when I first felt I had entered something worthwhile in my life. I was assisting some of these students with personal care and feeding, and it was the first time I was working around nurses. There weren't many of these clinicians, but they were known to everyone in the school, college and residential premises. They were buzzing around the place with high concentration and assertiveness. They worked in a language that wasn't translatable to me back then. But I knew they were kind, hard-working, and passionate people. I marvelled at their compassion, sympathy and empathy towards helping the students at their most vulnerable moments, and they really helped make it a place of sanctuary for them.

Never in a million years would the schoolboy me, in his football kit, have imagined that I'd eventually become a nurse. I didn't realise then that I'd find exactly what I'd searched for (minus being a professional footballer for Tottenham Hotspur); that nursing would be my true calling, with a sprinkling of other little projects, including writing, to get my creative juices flowing. What I've learnt over the years about nursing and my memoir writing is that they both go together well; it's about constantly tuning into your inner self and stepping into the shoes of others.

In current times, there are popular medical TV shows like *Grey's Anatomy* and *Scrubs*, and real-life programmes such as *24 Hours in A&E*. Books about the experiences of healthcare workers also enjoy great popularity, especially those by Adam Kay, an author who's achieved stardom after writing about his medical reflections as a gynaecological doctor. This tells me that there's a growing interest from the public to gain insight from the stories of medical professionals. In my writings as a community nurse focusing on the hardships and positivity that came from COVID-19, I believed there would be a big target audience of enthusiastic readers, as everyone can relate to that fearful period in our lives.

Community nursing, the career I eventually moulded myself into after being awarded my postgraduate diploma, remains quite hidden in the background of the National Health Service (NHS). I don't think many people know about the role of a community nurse, but I hope this book and my earlier memoir will raise awareness of this nursing field in non-medical readers. These writings go into depth about the diverse range of clinical skills, which are mandatory as a community nurse, demonstrating how unpredictable the job is from one day to the next, whilst following the essential guidance in our policies and protocols.

A statistic that struck a chord with me when writing my previous memoir came from a report in May 2019 from the Royal College of Nursing (RCN), which revealed that the number of district nurses had fallen by 43% over the past decade. Nurses in all areas are highly skilled health professionals that the nation cannot live without, and they get nowhere near the recognition they deserve. Even after the masses that stood and clapped in homage to the heroic efforts of the nurses in 2020, this statistic of district nurses has remained unchanged, if not worsened, despite how necessary this profession is in all communities.

Community nurses don't always know what type of person they'll visit or the environment they'll operate within. We see a broad scale of people with underlying health conditions of various ages (mostly over 65) and from all walks of life. We can see the bubbly, independent ones who are cheerful and have good family support networks. We can also see the severely frail, the dejected, the lonely, and those who are extremely dependent on their life-limiting conditions. We thrive in making a positive difference to people's lives, even when we add that extra comfort to those at death's door.

You'll find that this book focuses a lot of attention on tissue viability, particularly after being appointed the Enhanced Wound Care Nurse in one of the local community nursing teams. With the new specialised role, I've strived to look for ways to improve the management of chronic or hard-to-heal wounds, for example, pressure ulcers, lower limb diabetic ulcers or venous leg ulcers. As a British Journal of Nursing article pointed out, these categories of wounds are increasing year on year, in parallel with the ageing population and coupled with the rise in the incidence of prolonged high-risk conditions, including COVID-19, in recent times. You'll also notice from these diary entries that I repeatedly work with tissue viability nurses known as TVNs; experts in providing specialist evidence-based advice on treatment of complex and non-healing wounds.

Writing these memoirs has given me another purpose; to do something worthwhile, and receiving amazing feedback gave me confidence in testing the waters again by writing a further book. One of the other main reasons I've written these memoirs is to highlight how significant nurses are, not just in my separate field but in general. My hope in writing these books is to demonstrate how admirable it is to be so professional and resilient at what we do, despite how undervalued we've been, even during and after the dark days of the global pandemic. And why enough was enough for our demand in pay to be increased to what we deserve in an era that's been financially crippling for many.

Whatever you may think about nurses, remember that however good or bad our lives are, we've all been born, we're all going to be very unwell or injured (or both) at some point and we're all going to die. In most of these scenarios, you'll be cared for by a nurse in a hospital or at home if you're housebound. These people caring for you have been and will show you kindness, compassion and empathy. They don't discriminate. They visit people of all ages in homes, waiting rooms, corridors and wards. The rich and poor, the disabled and able-bodied, the blind or sighted, the physically or mentally ill, and people of all races and cultural upbringings. So, what I'm getting at is that we live up to the phrase, "If you save one life, you're a hero. Save 100 lives, and you're a nurse."

CHAPTER 1
A NEW YEAR WITH COVID STILL LURKING

Friday, 15th January 2021

I'm glad this new year hasn't been recognised as 'the year of the nurse.' No-one expected what would happen when that title was assigned to 2020 when our world changed not for the better, and when sanitiser became our closest friend. The year has started on a funny note, though. Well, today anyway, as the administration lady in charge of purchasing medical supplies in bulk needed to order lube that we use for clinical procedures like catheter changes. We were surprised this morning when we came into the office and saw a few boxes. I took one sachet out and realised that the boxes contained sachets of a different branded lube. This brand claims to spice up your sexual desires with your lover in the bedroom. It is safe to say that the administration lady was slightly embarrassed by her mishap. At least those in loving relationships have a treat for the weekend.

Thursday, 28th January 2021

I can often be mistaken as 'the doctor' when I visit a service user's home. Being called the doctor has happened in the past, either by the deranged patient or by the caregiver being on the phone with a patient's friend or relative. Even though we nurses are assertive and competent professionals, I still take these snippets of miscommunication as small compliments as it obviously shows that I present as someone self-assured and comfortable in their skin and because a doctor hardly ever attempts a home appointment nowadays, they anticipate that a male medic in blue will finally be the doctor that they've wanted to see.

Today was no exception, and to be fair, the visit where I was asked the question "Are you the doctor?" was from a patient expecting the duty doctor to evaluate their views and wishes while they can still make their own decisions despite their diagnosed dementia. But even after explaining myself as the clinician reviewing this patient's skin tear on her arm, I overheard the live-in carer say, "The doctor is here now to review Mary's Respect form," when she answered the phone to Mary's daughter.

During an introductory palliative visit, it's a good idea to check if the service user has a Respect form or if they'd consider one. The Respect form is assessed and completed by a GP (short for General Practitioner, and another term for a doctor registered at the patient's health centre). The Respect form records a patient's limit of care with their treatment preferences. It includes whether they'd still decide to be resuscitated in the event of a cardiac arrest, even though some ribs can be cracked if someone is providing pounding chest compressions on their delicate chest. They may not have any consciousness if they survive, bearing in mind the survival rates of CPR in community settings are no more than 10%. The patient's preferences will also include whether they still want to receive acute hospital care if they deteriorate, typically through infection and life-threatening sepsis. The Respect form can also state the preferred place of death.

Nonetheless, it makes me chuckle that I can be perceived as a doctor/GP. It's a shame that my pay doesn't reflect the misinterpretation, but I'd gladly decline their levels of demand and stress, especially in the busy hospital wards. You've only got to watch or read Adam Kay's tales from *This is Going to Hurt* to find that out.

When I hear these incorrect remarks, though, it makes me realise how people from older generations still struggle to understand that men can be nurses and women are doctors. It's not black and white anymore. Society has changed for the better in terms of equality.

Friday, 5th February 2021

About six months ago, we were visiting a lady called Beryl, who had cut a hole in her rugged settee so that she could urinate and defecate into it. She can use her very own toilet within the confines of her lounge. You may think it's just plain lazy, but it's simply an unfortunate case of self-neglect. Her life and family have flashed before her eyes, and she turned to alcohol and doesn't have much of an appetite anymore. At least she had the decency of placing incontinence pads around the hole to avoid contaminating the rest of her leather settee in faecal matter.

She still had one terrific lady in her life who lived three doors down the road from her. They were both local ladies from the village who worked together in their own bakery business when they were in their 20s. I guess the friend wanted to show loyalty to Beryl, a friendship that couldn't be broken, despite whatever has occurred until now, when they reached their mid-60s. Beryl's friend was the only one who still visited the home, and she let herself in with her own key to clean up the living room every few days, plus what lay below the hole of doom.

Unfortunately, Beryl became too cantankerous in our care to help heal her category two sacral wounds. On the final encounter, she ordered me and a healthcare assistant to leave her alone and never return. Beryl was assessed by a mental health professional that same week as having the capacity to make her own decisions, so we had no choice but to discharge her from our caseload and inform the doctor. Just before we did this, Beryl had also cancelled the package of care that we managed to organise. It covered her prepping for meals and medication, overseeing hygiene needs, doing regular skin checks of all bony prominences, and offering advice on pressure relief, such as standing up routinely in the daytime to relieve her bottom from further pressure damage.

None of us have heard any news from this lady since the discharge, not even a blood test request from the doctor. Occasionally, I think about people like her who were discharged with major vulnerabilities. I wonder what's become of her. Is she still wallowing in her mess on the settee, wasting away in one room of a spacious bungalow? Does her loyal friend still visit her? Has she died of malnourishment, an infection, a disease, or COVID? Has she made a miraculous turnaround in her life with improved health and finding some happiness again, which she once had in previous work, friendship, marriage, and family life? Many of these unanswered questions stir around mine and my colleagues' minds now and again, hoping that whatever has happened to "so-and-so" has been positive and not saddening or disastrous.

Friday, 26th February 2021

When a service user presents with a red discoloured patch of skin on a bony prominence of their body that does not change colour when pressed, it's our duty as community nurses to investigate other holistic aspects. This becomes an absolute necessity if they develop higher categories of pressure damage, when open wounds need treating with dressings. It's also our duty to risk assess their setup at home and ensure they're using the most appropriate equipment to help avoid deterioration of existing pressure ulcers and prevent the possibility of them developing or redeveloping. We can review patients' needs for pressure-relieving cushions if they spend a lot of time sitting in chairs which may have firm, uncomfortable seating. Another piece of equipment that we must pay close attention to is the type of mattress on the bed. Any ordinary divan mattress will be no good for someone who's showing a mild score or higher for developing pressure damage to their skin on the risk assessment tool. For example, someone malnourished and spending longer hours in bed compared to the average person will have a higher risk of bed sores.

When we analyse pressure-relieving mattresses, the cheapest version of these is the Propad foam mattress overlay, only costing the NHS £65, and these should be used solely for patients who are at mild-to-moderate risk of pressure damage. Next on the list is the Mercury soft-form mattress, made of a memory foam material, and it's suitable for patients with a greater chance of developing pressure injuries and with a weight limit of 22 stone, which will cost the NHS £152 to be loaned out. Then there's the Hybrid mattress, which can be used with the equivalent quality of a Mercury foam mattress, but with a pump installed into this mattress, it can transform into an air-flow mattress for added pressure relief. The Hybrid mattress, in total, will cost the NHS £500 per service user, and they can be useful for a patient in a remote area who may be at risk of a power cut. With the air-flow version of these in mind, operating on a one-in-three-cell inflation cycle, they should be ordered for those with a very high chance of getting bed sores. The most enhanced mattress is the Quattro Plus air-flow system mattress, costing £900 on loan and requires a pump to operate on a one-in-four cell cycle, and these mattresses should be prescribed for the treatment and prevention of pressure ulcers.

Most of our community patients spend their days lying in bed or sitting in a chair. Therefore, it's paramount that cushions and mattresses (the two main pieces of equipment in their lives) have the optimum level of comfort and pressure-relieving qualities to suit each individual. This is only possible with risk assessments from the professionals involved in the patient's multi-disciplinary team. A lot of the time, the risk assessments and decision-making for ordering equipment or referring to another type of specialised care will come down to the community nurses. This is because they're usually the first point of call to the initial presenting problem of a pressure injury somewhere on the body, characteristically on the bottom, spine or heels, and this already falls under a nursing need to improve the skin integrity of the vulnerable and damaged areas on the body.

When treating morbidly obese people, I refer to them as plus-sized or bariatric individuals. I've been complimented on this as a polite form of terminology. Karen was a lady I visited today who falls within the plus-sized category. She was recently discharged from hospital with resolved bowel obstruction, and she's been weighed at 220 kilograms. Over time, she's taken to her privately purchased, all-singing and dancing bariatric bed with incline features and with that and the memory foam mattress in place, it cost £7,500. We've been referred to treat Karen's wounds on her sacrum, which split open in the hospital. Our wound care regime will rely on the help of the carers visiting four times a day and her hardworking husband to not only meet all of Karen's activities of daily living, such as dressing and feeding her, but also to change her incontinence pads on each visit, with two-people operating these interventions each time with the assistance of slide sheets to alleviate the strain on our backs when turning her. We've caught the wounds early with merely the top layer of skin removed, but the need for an enhanced air-flow mattress screams out to me, much to Karen and her husband's resentment because they forked out money for equipment that they thought would set her for life. Even though I said I was hopeful to replace the current mattress with one that was

NHS-funded, there were still logistical issues regarding how a new air-flow mattress would be installed on Karen's bed. Karen would need to be hoisted for a start, which hadn't been risk-assessed in the community by the occupational therapists. She'd also need to sit in her armchair temporarily while the mattress is installed and inflated by the technician, something she hasn't been used to for several years. As well as that, there's limited space in her bedroom to manoeuvre a mobile hoist and switch the large-scaled mattresses in one fell swoop.

However you categorise these patients, there is a clear need for closer professional discussions and examinations when identifiable problems occur at their homes. In pressure ulcer awareness training, I learned that plus-sized people are two times more likely to develop pressure injuries compared to other people. Therefore, it's important to be aware of poorly fitting equipment. Sometimes, we need to refer to the occupational therapists or the redistribution service to search for and order the most appropriate appliances that offer the best weight distribution and that, when installed, will work effectively. This is especially important before we discharge a service user because we don't want to have bigger fish to fry further down the line. To emphasise this fact, I remember a patient being re-referred to us with a hole on the base of their spine due to one of the inflated panels of their mattress becoming deflated, meaning the patient's back was essentially lying on an unforgiving plank of wood from the base of the bed. Perhaps there were faults with the mattress before discharge; we wouldn't know unless we did a final risk assessment, but we also need to put our trust in our patients to promptly speak out concerns about something within our remit.

There's an increasing prevalence of obesity, the primary factor driving the upsurge of the global market for bariatric beds. According to the World Health Organisation (WHO), obesity has nearly tripled since 1975, and in 2016, over 1.9 billion adults 18 years and older were overweight; of these, over 650 million were obese. I'm confident these statistics have worsened since then, and the population of plus-sized people is expected to grow as the decades go by because of society and lifestyle changes. We can order groceries, dinners and anything we need with the touch of a few buttons on our smartphones, and they come straight to our door. There's less need to walk anywhere, and the younger generations stay indoors and entertained by social media and video games. More people are overindulging in their favourite fast foods, which are shoved in our faces on TV with subliminal messages everywhere to *consume*, and because of less social interaction, people are becoming less body conscious. They can make themselves look flattering by the filters on their camera phone and the angle at which they point it.

In my additional responsibility as an equipment prescriber, I'm going to need to be increasingly mindful to select an appliance for not only the protection of skin integrity for plus-sized individuals like Karen but also to enable them to perform their daily activities and maintain a degree of independence and quality of life. Caregivers and nurses are people the NHS and agencies within the health and social care sector desperately rely on; however, when they assist with medical interventions and these everyday tasks, they can increase the possibility of musculoskeletal injuries. So, it's not just about promoting the health and well-being of our patients that we focus on when providing these risk assessments. It's just as critical to consider our own welfare.

CHAPTER 2
ONE FINAL BREATH

Wednesday, 17th March 2021

I visited 95-year-old Chester today, who was actively dying, as notified by the palliative nurse who reviewed them yesterday. Following on from the Trust's end-of-life care strategy and with advanced care planning started in the early phase, I was now at the stage of planning on replenishing Chester's syringe driver with the exact measurements of oxycodone and midazolam as he seemed to have remained at a steady, therapeutic yet semi-conscious level for the past two days. The quivering and whimpering have now subsided. In many situations, nurses are there when the last breath is taken, and nurses are also there when the first breath is taken, particularly in the labour wards. As humans, we're well adapted to celebrating one's birth, but from a nursing standpoint, it's just as important to find comfort in death, and this is no different in Chester's case.

Today, the young female Gambian carer greeted me in the home and assured me that Chester was calm overnight. He was the same gentleman lying flat on his back in the bed, his mouth wide open and his eyes also open but with a glazed, vacant stare towards the ceiling. His face and hands had become much paler since I last saw him on the urgent call-out on Monday night, when he kept wandering out of bed without his zimmer frame and shouting inaudible garbage at the caregiver. The palliative medications have had a great effect on Chester in recent days. Still, he's rapidly deteriorated, no thanks to his fierce metastatic cancer of the kidneys, which we knew had spread to his liver. The surface of the tongue and roof of the mouth looked rough and dry like orange sandpaper in the warm yellow ray of sun shining over him this morning.

I advised the carer to moisten Chester's dry mouth with a baby toothbrush dipped in water. She did this for a couple of minutes while Chester was upright. Just in case he needed to give a weak swallow. Moments later, while I was preparing Chester's medications to replenish the syringe driver, the caregiver was concerned about his breathing. There were increasingly sizeable delays in his breaths. The first interval I observed was about five seconds, then eight seconds in the next breath and then 12 seconds in the breath that followed. These were apparent features of what practitioners call Cheyne-stokes breathing. With each faint and shallow inhalation, the head and neck simultaneously tilted away from the pillow. His mouth was still wide open, and glassy eyes still gazing ahead. It was the body's way of shutting down.

"Don't worry, Hazel, he's comfortable," I say to his frail four-foot-eight wife, who intently watches on with sadness in her armchair opposite the hospital bed in the living room.

"Do you want to go into the conservatory? Your garden looks lovely on a day like today." "Yes, I think I will," Hazel says, half-smiling. She slowly places on her sun hat, grabs today's newspaper in one hand and the wooden walking stick in the other, and trudges through to the kitchen and into the conservatory whilst staring at the floor the whole time until she sits on the wicker chair. I then sit back in the kitchen chair and prepare the vials of medication lined up on the table.

Moments later, the live-in carer looks at me in panic, saying, "I think he's gone." I then rush into the living room and observe Chester just as intently as the carer has done for the past 20 minutes. I also agree that Chester has taken his final breath of life. This is the first time someone has died in front of me. It's a good job that this was an anticipated death, too, whereby the doctor visited the patient within two weeks, and both the family members and the GP were aware that Chester was expected to die.

Fortunately, I had a form on me to complete the verification of death, which I've been competent in doing for nearly a year. I've provided this duty on several occasions, but today was different. Unlike the other incidents, Chester had literally just died, and it gave me a bit of an eery chill down my spine that he may not be completely lifeless. My mind was trying to play tricks on me. I sometimes wondered whether I saw his chest rise slightly or his lips and arms twitching.

Nonetheless, I did the necessary inspections to verify clinical signs of life. A lack of spontaneous activity? Absolutely yes. An absence of respiration? I get my stethoscope out and tap on the central areas of the chest, and I cannot hear activity from the airways. So, yes. An absence of carotid pulse or heart sounds? I check for several seconds for a pulse on the wrist and feel nothing. No response to physical stimuli? I was nervous the gentleman might flinch at this one because it would make any other living person jump from a natural sleep. I firmly squeezed the trapeze muscle a couple of times. No response. Are pupils not responding to light? For this, I bring out my pen torch, and with my gloved index finger, I push up the left eyelid to fully see the eye. I shine the light on the pupil, and there's no change in size. I also do this with the right eye, and the pupil has no dilation. Yet another tick to a question. After five minutes, I repeat all the checks, and it's the same outcome. I can confirm that Chester died at 10:35 a.m., and the form is now ready for the doctor's certification. I go into the conservatory and break the news to Hazel, who's in the carer's company.

"I'm sorry, Hazel, but Chester has now died." I put an arm around her shoulder.

"It's okay. I know he was at peace. He looked peaceful to me, and that's all we can have hoped for, isn't it... We all have to go somewhere, don't we? It's just part of life." My heart melted after Hazel's sweet little speech. She took the loss so well at the most sensitive stage and was so accepting. It seemed like she'd prepared herself all week for this moment. But I could see the eyes beginning to lubricate, and she gently rose from her seat and with her hunched physique, she crept back into the living room to see Chester one last time, following a 65-year marriage.

With that, the live-in carer calls her phone as if her life depended on it. At the same time, I calmly contact the nurse on shift and tell them to inform the local surgery of Chester's passing, and then I take a photo of the verification form as a copy, which I'll use to show the GP later in an email. Just after I do that, I get the carer's phone shoved in my face, saying that the hospice team wants a word. When I answer, I get Lydia, the palliative nurse, asking me if everything's okay. I said, "Well, apart from the patient dying, we're doing okay."

She replied, "Please don't call for an ambulance when an end-of-life patient has had an expected death."

In response, I said, "Of course not."

Lydia then says, "Well, please tell the carer that because that's what she wants to do." I then quickly end the call and rush into the lounge because I can see the carer using the patient's house phone.

"No! Please don't call for an ambulance!" I say, reluctantly raising my voice in such a delicate situation. The caregiver then passes the landline phone to me, shamefaced. I glance back in bewilderment and disappointment to resemble a teacher looking at their star pupil who royally fucked up their exam. I then had to apologise to the local ambulance service for wasting a few precious minutes of their time and briefly explain the reasons why with some embarrassment.

The niece is the next of kin and the only family member looking out for this couple because Chester and Hazel never had children. The niece loved her auntie and uncle because she came to the door minutes after being informed with a bright pink sports top and black leggings. She went straight over to Hazel with a huge hug, and Hazel finally released her emotions.

Shortly after their welcomed embrace, the niece turned to me with red, tearful eyes and mascara running down both cheeks. She giggled, "I knew going to Pilates this morning was a bad idea. I left the sports hall without warning when the carer told me the news." She said "sorry" to Hazel, but I'm sure Hazel didn't mind because she absolutely adores her niece and bent over backwards for the couple. The niece was the one who organised a package of care when she knew the couple's mobility was declining and management of their activities of daily living was becoming a problem. And she's been the *eyes and ears* for the community nurses, doctor and hospice teams to discuss any concerns about Chester's symptoms and be the one to collect more medication from the pharmacy when we were close to running out. One of her final tasks for Chester was to contact the local funeral directors to attend to the body and prepare the care after death.

Just as she made that call, I thought, "shit, this gentleman has still got two medical devices attached to his body and one of them is infusing medication unnecessarily," which was utterly undignified.

I politely asked the carer to assist me with sorting out Chester, who seemed to be on tenterhooks after her calamity. We raised the hospital bed to the carer's shorter waistline and gently rolled Chester on both sides to remove his pyjama bottoms and the incontinence pad. While doing this, I intuitively said a few words to Chester as if he was still alive.

"Okay, Chester, I'm just going to stop the syringe driver and remove it from your left thigh now.

"Hmm... what did you say?" The carer muttered with a puzzled look to me.

"Oh, I was just talking to Chester." The carer then opens her mouth slightly, glancing at me with bemusement as if I'm a bloody moron talking to a dead person. To me, this was a natural reaction as a nurse. Ever since I had my first episode of last offices in a hospital placement during my student days, I was told by the senior nurses to treat the individual with absolute dignity and respect. If family members are present, it's comforting for them to know that you're taking such lovely care of their loved one's body. It's only how Chester wanted to be treated anyway, right? I was then perturbed about whether the carer had enough valuable experience for their duties.

For the next part, I warned the wife and niece that they probably would want to leave the room, and they kindly did because I was about to remove Chester's urethral catheter, which was inserted by the palliative nurse yesterday. We often catheterise patients in end-of-life care who are showing signs of agitation. One of the reasons for their agitation could be that their body is struggling to void urine. Therefore, this causes urine to be stored in the bladder and irritates the muscle from the acidity of the content. The patient instinctively tries to leave the bed to go to the toilet. This proved another good solution for Chester, and surprisingly, he had 250 millilitres of amber-coloured urine in his catheter bag despite not actively drinking in the last three days.

I then opened a 10-millilitre syringe onto a sterile drape lying beside the patient on his bed and as I was about to deflate the balloon, the carer said, "Nope. I can't see this. I'm going next door, too."

Just as I was starting to deflate the balloon, the doorbell rang. It was two members of the funeral service.

I thought to myself, "Fuck. What will they think of me removing a catheter in the middle of the lounge when they were informed the body was ready to collect?" The carer then walked over to the front door. I had to apologise as the funeral directors walked across the room to speak with the niece in the kitchen to discuss plans with the undertakers and the funeral service. Then as the caregiver walked past me, I was removing the tip of the catheter from the penis.

"Nope. Nope. Nope." The carer said whilst placing both hands out parallel to eye level. What did she think I was going to do? Squirt her with a water pistol, like I'd have done if I was 10 again. After what she saw, she ran upstairs to throw up in the bathroom.

After disposing of the waste from the catheter removal, I carefully pulled up Chester's trouser bottoms again and tucked him into bed with uncreased bedsheets. My job was almost done.

"All finished now, Chester," I say after completing the clinical procedure. I then confirmed with the funeral director that I was happy for them to continue the care after death. I notified the niece that all medications belonging to Chester need to be returned to the pharmacy and to contact the local equipment stores about collecting all items loaned out to Chester. I make her and Hazel aware that they can interact with the GP and the hospice service for advice and options if they need support with bereavement.

The niece replied, "I'm more concerned that Hazel will be alone now. I know the live-in carer was assigned for Chester, but I will contact the agency and see if I can keep the carer on for another week until I can find something more sustainable. After all, I'm paying for this privately." What such a caring thing to say, I thought to myself.

"It will likely be a care home that Hazel will need next." She whispered subtly in my ear, avoiding any added distress for Hazel at such a difficult time. I then gave my heartfelt condolences to the family members, and they sent their gratitude to me and the outstanding community services that helped Chester through the terminal phase.

For uni students training to become nurses, the sciences of chemistry, biology, and physics, are imperative. When I was a student at the University of Southampton, they'd spend hours learning about the anatomy and physiology of how the body works. They'll be learning about the pharmacology of how a multitude of medicines work with their possible side effects. As much as this is all paramount in becoming a competent and confident practitioner, it's only when you're operating as a qualified nurse you understand that the philosophy, psychology and ethics of a nurse hold far greater weight. This episode of care today correlates to the three latter aspects, which are meaningful for the patients we care for and the colleagues we work alongside during our careers.

CHAPTER 3
A DISCONNECTED FAMILY

Saturday, 3rd April 2021

Ian Pete OBE, who's also Editor in Chief for the British Journal of Nursing, has stated in an article that in England and Wales the population continues to age, and the 2021 Census results confirm there are more people than ever before in the older age groups; over 11 million people. To put that into perspective, that's 18.6% of the total population aged 65 years or older, in contrast to 16.4% at the time of the earlier Census in 2011. It comprised of over half a million (527,900) people at least 90 years of age, per the Office for National Statistics in 2022.

Living longer is something that should be celebrated as our ageing population brings with it opportunities. Older people can make valuable contributions to societies and the economy. For example, through continued employment, providing informal caregiving for grandchildren, parents and other relatives and they can contribute by volunteering. As people age, however, the probability of becoming ill and frail increases, resulting in a greater need for health and social care with a risk of developing several long-term conditions. It can include neurological diseases such as dementia.

It was my turn to have weekend duties. I was visiting service users outside my team's area who I was unaware of, reducing the weekend strain of a struggling neighbouring team. On one of my visits, I was greeted by a 65-year-old called Barry, who has type two diabetes and a recent diagnosis of vascular dementia, and I couldn't help but see a connection to the meaning of Ian Pete's article and this gentleman's age-related deterioration. Barry requires daily blood glucose monitoring and prepping his long-acting insulin at the precise dose as prescribed before he attaches the needle, inserts it into the subcutaneous tissue of the tummy and self-administers the injection. Even though it was morning when I saw him, he had a beef stew bubbling on the stove, which he said he'll have a portion of as an early lunch after I leave. He added that he'll get several extra servings from the stew for the week ahead. It had a lovely, homely aroma, and Barry said he's always enjoyed cooking. I'm sure it would've tasted delicious, and my tummy agreed with a rumble.

After the necessary interventions were completed on the visit, Barry really opened up to me about his life as he now knows it. He had a chirpiness to him to begin with, grinning at the thought that he could potter around his garden later with a warm, sunny spring afternoon in the forecast. But I did notice that his face changed to a less cheerful one later in our conversation. I could sense a feeling of desolation in his eyes, and I felt that he wanted to have a man-to-man chat, pouring out part of his soul to me.

The tender part of the conversation started with him saying that he was an engineer by trade, and through his experience, he went from novice to expert for British Telecom. He was regularly called up for advice by the apprentices, even in out-of-hour periods. Barry then went on to say that he has a partner. I didn't get round to asking if they were married, but Barry said she lives in a house in Portsmouth rather than his flat 20 miles away. They decided to part ways when Barry was diagnosed with dementia, and he found himself being out of his normal character. He'd go to the shops and forget what he intended to buy. Not only that, but he failed to dress appropriately over the recent winter we had. Instead of trousers, jumpers, and coats, he'd wear shorts and a t-shirt or go straight out in his dressing gown and slippers after waking up for the day. Barry was also becoming verbally aggressive towards his partner, as unpleasant characteristics manifested since his diagnosis. Is this simply a result of damage to the brain, or did frustration in the transformation of Barry's mental health contribute to his regretful actions that didn't help with their split? Again, this wasn't spoken about in any detail, and I could see that this topic was starting to touch on Barry's emotions.

Besides that, Barry pushed that shame aside and assured me he and his partner were still together. They still have love for each other. An eternal bond. He said he sees her for a few days every couple of weeks. He usually stays at her house in Portsmouth and meets her at the train station. Over the few days together, the partner can assist in managing his diabetic care.

They have a daughter, who's 25 years old, and unfortunately, she has Dandy-Walker syndrome. I wasn't aware of this rare condition before today, but Barry informed me that it's when one of the lobes in the brain is missing. It's a cystic malformation in the cerebellum, to be precise. This malformation blocks the cerebrospinal fluid from exiting the brain, consequently increasing intracranial pressure and affecting the individual's motor skills, such as walking. No matter how upsetting it is that the daughter has a compromised life and perhaps a shortened life expectancy, Barry still spoke about her with such pride. He explained that she takes life in her stride and gets on well with him and his partner. He knows this because when she's insulting someone, that means she likes that person, and she predictably says to Barry when they first meet: "Are you not dead yet?" He added that she's very good with the English language and admirably she's written articles for the local newspaper.

Barry then turns his compliments toward his partner and says she has a successful career as a mental health professional. In her current leadership role, she's working in prisons, supporting a group of scarred youths. Just as he was in the engineering trade, the partner is an expert in her field, and she's often invited to be a speaker for university cohorts in mental health courses. From a more personal standpoint, she's moulded herself into the perfect mother and role model for her daughter, which is comforting for Barry, and he doesn't feel so bad being a distant father figure.

Despite Barry's slightly restricted lifestyle nowadays, I could still see a degree of contentment. He still has plenty of independence. Even though he has domiciliary care once a day, he still cooks for himself, does the day-to-day activities inside his flat, and does gardening when the weather is nice.

On the other hand, he doesn't know how long he has this level of independence for. He's already lost much of his life at the house with his partner and child, and he realises he will lose more parts of his life when his dementia progresses. I could tell he was apprehensive about his future at the end of our conversation. He worries about when he'll have to give up the flat and when a care home is the next stage. He thanked me for seeing him today, but when we said goodbye at the front door, I couldn't help noticing the glint of sadness in his eyes.

CHAPTER 4
EXTRA PENNIES ON THE ROAD

Tuesday, 27th April 2021

Taking digital images of patient's wounds and uploading them onto our clinical database is essential for our visual records. They're uploaded directly from our encrypted apps on the work phones. Under the Data Protection Act, it's important we gain consent before doing so and make sure the patients are fully aware of the rationale for taking wound photos, which are to show any noticeable changes during wound treatment or signs of skin deterioration or the rarity of being used for research purposes and case studies. It can reassure them that we won't publish images of their bottom sores on our social media pages or the front page of News of the World.

There's a lady who has a long-standing wound on her leg, and with each visit, she's requesting a £10 fee for each photo we take of her leg before the many dressing changes are provided. The leg is getting somewhat famous now with all the attention it's having from the paparazzi of nurses. If we'd accepted her charges, she'd have become quite a wealthy lady this summer.

Saturday, 1st May 2021

At last, our Trust has increased our fuel allowance, although at this rate, with the oil prices rising, we may have to take drastic measures and go back to using bikes. But when I think I do an average of 30 business miles a day in my car, imagine the pulsating veins in my achy thighs as I pedal up those hills with hefty belongings. There's a high chance that our wheels would be nicked, plus you'd need a trailer with all the supplies we carry. The amount of extra time for travelling that we'd need isn't worth thinking about. There'll be no time to write our progress notes in the office as we'll be cycling most of the day in our vast geographical areas. And with the number of potholes building up on the roads now, it'll surely be far too dangerous and impractical when you're the one with the student for the day. *Call the Midwife* is probably the TV show with the closest similarities to district nursing, despite the outdatedness; however, those ladies you see on their bikes in the series represent a time in history that's not logistically feasible to return to.

Wednesday, 5th May 2021

A student nurse almost passed out on one of my visits today after watching me perform a routine suprapubic catheter change. Unlike the typical urinary catheter, that carries urine from the bladder and through the urethra and the opening of the penis or vagina, suprapubic versions are inserted into the lower abdomen and into the bladder to drain urine. As mentioned in my previous book, suprapubic catheters are usually considered an alternative if there are too many complications with urethral catheters.

Today's suprapubic catheter change was performed on a young female patient, who yelps every time the catheter is removed and inserted, but this is more of a coping mechanism for her rather than displaying discomfort. Before I started, the student told me that she hadn't seen a suprapubic catheter site before, and it probably didn't help that the catheter site was unusual looking, presenting with over-granulation (proud-flesh raised above the wound margins). Over-granulation can be caused by irritation, commonly the rubbing of the catheter tubing, thus causing the skin to over-heal and preventing epithelialisation from happening. The epithelial tissue is the last stage of wound healing when new healthy tissue has reformed. Unlike epithelial tissue, over-granulation isn't something we want to see. It can bleed easily, and because infection can be the other cause, anti-microbial dressings can be another form of treatment. In this patient's case, she's having her site treated with a steroid cream, which can heal the over-granulation by bringing down the inflammation.

To someone not used to the clinical intervention of changing a suprapubic catheter, it may look somewhat malicious, especially with the flashback of bloodstained urine trickling through the tubing by the end. I peered over at the silent student, about to ask her if she had any questions about what she just saw. But the young student's face turned pale; her eyes were dilated as she froze and looked up at the ceiling. She had her hands clenched on the side rail of the patient's hospital bed to keep her balance, but she started to sway from side to side, and I was concerned she might collapse at any second.

I left the sterile field I was working on, leapt across the room, and carefully supported the student out of the home as if she were a vulnerable patient about to take the taxi to a clinic appointment. The patient's mother kindly placed a chair outside and gave the student a glass of water, and I let her sit and relax for a short while until I packed up and said my goodbyes to the patient. The student nurse was embarrassed and kept saying sorry for how she reacted. She had nothing to apologise about. I was sorry not to prewarn her enough about the medical intervention, and from now on, when a newcomer is shadowing me, I'll provide an introduction before I undertake any invasive treatments or gruesome wound care.

Wednesday, 19th May 2021

I undertook a blood test for a gentleman sitting in their study room. In a phlebotomist role for a visit, I was taking the blood from one of the veins on the antecubital fossa, located on the opposite side of the elbow. These veins are most suitable for phlebotomy as they tend to be more visible here, especially once using the tourniquet, normally fastened 10 centimetres above the attempted vein and is applied to help find the veins and used for a maximum time of 60 seconds as anything above this time increases the risk of the blood supply being cut off. On this topic, we nurses have a guilty obsession with observing people's veins. It could be a family member at home or a random person in the public. I could be looking at their arms queueing up in the supermarket and thinking, "Cor! They've got a juicy, springy vein right there. I could easily get blood through a needle in that one!"

Suppose the familiar veins are difficult to find or the service user is stingy with their blood. In that case, we can consider the alternative site, which is the thinner veins on the back of the hand, with a higher chance of triggering pain on needle insertion. Reluctant veins can also occur from anxiety, causing temporarily increased blood pressure to narrow the blood vessels, which is why I typically have a laid-back approach to the patient on these visits, putting their mind at ease by making small talk about life and even getting them to turn their head away until I start my needle poking with a "sharp scratch." The patient's health can also influence whether I'll get their blood. If they're malnourished or dehydrated, this can be mission impossible with blood sampling. We should urge the patient to improve their fluid intake and ensure they warm themselves up with a hot water bottle or blanket in the cooler months to avoid the veins constricting.

We're taught only to have a maximum of two attempts with blood-taking. Usually, it's best to use two attempts in one arm and leave a spare arm for another clinician to have a go if unsuccessful, much to the patient's disgust, who won't want to be used as a human pin cushion.

On today's visit, instead of any of the above considerations before taking blood, there was a completely new preparation method. I went into the lounge to put down my supplies, and when I returned to see the patient and check the veins in his arms, he was on his knees. I was unsettled that he'd taken a funny turn and asked if he was OK, and I was willing to help him sit back in his chair. The gentleman said he was fine; with that, he went on all fours in dog mode. I was bemused at this point and turned to the little wife, who was also frail with a hunched back but was the more independent of the two. She said so casually, "Oh, it's fine. He will crawl now." With that, the gentleman crawled into the other room for his blood test like a giant toddler. The wife added, "he does this sometimes because it's much quicker than when he walks with his trolley."

To give him his due, he was a decent crawler for a mid-80-year-old, and he could manoeuvre himself into a seat on the settee with no problems. After taking the blood test, I checked his knees, and there was no sign of carpet burns, hopefully indicating that he doesn't do this sort of thing too often. Otherwise, he'll be referred to the physios to encourage him to walk more.

Friday, 28th May 2021

The team are currently visiting a lady of 38 years old in the local community hospital ward. She's been diagnosed with a prolapsed lumbar intervertebral disc, and due to this, she has nil feeling in her rectum. Therefore, daily rectal stimulation is a requirement to have her bowels open when sitting on the commode later in the day. This is the primary reason we're visiting this poor soul until she finds accommodation suitable to support her living elsewhere, with faculties that she needs, such as a wet room and walk-in shower. How the back injury started in the first place sounded horrendous. It was caused by a car accident five years previously. She sat in the back seat as a passenger, and the car was hit by a lorry on their way to a music festival, and the driver and passenger in the front seats were killed outright. She then required surgery, the removal of a disk in the spine. She's had altered sensation in her legs since then, and up until now, she's spent four months in a general hospital due to severe constipation and bowel obstruction.

Plato, an ancient Greek philosopher, rightly stated, "Be kind, for everyone you meet is fighting a battle." This lady is understandably facing personal battles, in a physical sense, and she's been left with mental health problems. She suffers from regular episodes of anxiety and panic attacks. She wondered how her life had been turned upside down due to events that should never have happened.

Nevertheless, horrific events you'd never imagine in your worst nightmares do occur. They can still become a reality for many who are extremely unfortunate. If that weren't bad enough, she told me today that she heard of three people she knew who died in quick succession recently. She told me she felt sad that she wouldn't be able to attend their funerals, which impacted her psychological well-being following her traffic accident. All I could do was sympathise with her before providing the slightly awkward bowel care with the sheepish healthcare assistant, as my chaperone, standing next to me. All I can do is ponder how strong-willed one must be to be left with a crippling existence of health complications and a sprinkling of stress and sorrow. Shit after shit to deal with, if you pardon the pun.

CHAPTER 5
A CHALLENGING LIFE WITH CHRONIC LEG OEDEMA

I'll start this chapter by mentioning that oedema is a fancy medical word for swelling and for a 54-year-old gentleman we've been re-referred to, this swelling is in the form of chronic lymphedema, which has worsened due to absences of compression therapy to their legs. Archie lives with his wife in a one-bedroom apartment. Due to Archie's severe lymphedema, alongside obesity and a stroke in 2019, Archie has found it challenging to get from room to room. Consequently, he's confined to the lounge area and just about managing to use the bathroom. Archie recently had a fall at the apartment, resulting in five paramedics supporting him up from the floor. Yep, he's that much of a plus-sized gentleman and wins the award for the most enormous legs I've ever seen. As we've known from this gentleman numerous times before, he's challenging when it comes to complying with our advice, which is why we discharged him from the caseload a year ago. Still, the concerned registered doctor brought Archie to our attention again, stating that the legs had become alarmingly swollen and sore. Just imagine two long balloons for the lower legs, two larger balloons of the same shape for the thighs and a couple of rounded balloons for the feet and imagine them being inflated so much that they might burst at any given second. That's what Archie's legs and feet looked like in the referral photo.

As explained in my previous book, a comprehensive Doppler assessment should be undertaken for oedematous or ulcerated legs or a combination of both. We couldn't provide a Doppler on Archie, though, because it relies on legs to be at heart level, but for Archie, his recliner chair cannot lay him into a supine position. He's been risk assessed by the occupational therapists as being unsafe to waddle and shuffle himself through the narrow gaps of the bedroom next door for a transfer in on the king-size bed that only the wife can enjoy. Dopplers have been used for vascular studies since the 1960s to examine the arterial blood flow of the lower limbs. Using the Doppler, we can determine the differential diagnosis of the leg ulceration. If the readings are in the normal range, that'll determine no arterial problems, and instead, the issues have less severity and are venous-related.

Arterial concerns in the legs include cramping pains in the calves at rest but generally when walking. This is known as intermittent claudication, which occurs because of muscle ischaemia. It cannot be accurately assessed in Archie's situation because his mobility has significantly reduced. Yet, other features of legs threatened by arterial complications include thin, shiny, hairless skin and a cold temperature, particularly in the feet, with differences in skin colour, such as blueness or paleness on elevation, compared to non-problematic lower limbs. These problems can escalate to signs of life-threatening ischaemia, and it's deemed unsafe to apply compression to limbs where there's identified ischaemia because it may occlude the arterial blood flow, decreasing limb perfusion, and resulting in a spread of necrosis, leading to amputation and even death.

It can be considered that the nurse's clinical judgement is more important than the outcome of a vascular test using a Doppler machine. I say this because when I spent the day at a vascular clinic at the local general hospital, the vascular consultant was evaluating patients with awfully oedematous and mishappened legs, and they decided that it was imperative for these patients to go into compression therapy treatments with some straightforward checks. They referred to their clinical judgement because they said the official calculated readings from a Doppler will primarily determine the arterial status. The consultant had no qualms with this because they felt that the peripheral pulses in the feet were palpable, the temperatures in the legs and feet were normal, the sensations in the feet were satisfactory, and the capillary refill in the toes was under two seconds when the skin was pressed. The consultant still inspected the pedal and tibial pulses of the feet with the Doppler probe. At the same time, the patients sat out in their chairs, and in all the cases where the pulses were identifiable, they were happy regardless of how clear the pulses sounded because the oedema may have also masked the strength of the pulse sounds. The clinicians who assessed Archie recently were satisfied with their knowledgeable checks, as they were last year, and strong compression therapy remains necessary on Archie's legs.

Wednesday, 7th April 2021

Archie is extremely worried about having a fall at home again, which would lead to the same ordeal as the other week, and there's a concern that transfers out of his recliner chair in the lounge are adding to the risk of a fall. With no surprise, Archie had blamed the compression bandage (that we've trialled for two weeks) for the cause of his latest fall.

There's a specific method on how to apply lymphedema compression bandaging, and it's the main form of treatment to reduce chronic leg oedema, but Archie won't allow for this to resume. The thigh-length stockings we ordered for Archie last year still miraculously fit both legs. He's agreed for these to be worn again, but the material is a mild form of compression, and it's been over-stretched with its elasticity as the leg circumferences are evidently greater than last year.

Nonetheless, Archie felt that the compression bandaging made it more difficult to get out of his riser-recliner chair because his legs felt even heavier and clumpier with it in situ and because of that inconvenience, he got the carer and his wife to cut it all off his legs before today's visit. He was adamant that he'll only wear compression hosiery from now on.

Wednesday, 28th April 2021

I organised for one of the local tissue viability nurses (TVNs) to come out with me today. Scarlett, the eccentric and ill-educated wife (when it comes to healthcare, anyway), opened the door for us today, and she had pent-up emotions and had a lot of things to get off her chest immediately. She said straight away that she believed Archie needed to go to the hospital to have a drain fitted to his legs to suck out the fluid, and she's been told this has been done before, and the sole reason why it won't happen is due to the NHS not wanting to pay for it. "It's because the NHS doesn't want to afford that treatment," she voiced abruptly before storming into the kitchen.

These accusations irritated the TVN, especially when Scarlett doesn't seem to take on board our service's recommendations historically and has tendencies to zone out and move into another room when she has nothing else to say. When Scarlett returned to the room today, the TVN explained to her (reiterating from a previous visit) that Archie had lymphedema. This lifelong condition must be managed with compression therapy. Scarlett remained fed up with receiving different information. Still, she did admit that her (outrageous) comments today came from a friend she bumped into at the newsagents and not from a qualified health professional. The TVN insisted that she shouldn't be listening to people who don't have knowledge of medical conditions.

Archie categorically refused to have compression bandages reapplied in spite of the professional advice, that this is the main way of reducing his lower limb oedema. As an alternative, we suggested to Archie that we re-measure his legs and thighs for customised compression hosiery but that this wouldn't lessen the severity of his build-up of lymph fluid. Wearing these stockings will only maintain the size of the legs as we see them now, and he'll need to wear them daily to halt his condition worsening. Archie seemed content to proceed with this alternative but denied us removing his current stockings to measure for the new hosiery. The TVN wasn't happy to use the measuring tape over these garments, as it could easily lead to inaccuracy of circumference measurements, avoiding around £580 of the NHS budget being potentially wasted for one pair of thigh-length made-to-measure stockings in the style that

Archie would require. That's the existing cost for just one set of these specialised garments that wouldn't be good to anyone unless they were used as giant leg warmers or perhaps a sleeping bag for a small child. The motive for Archie declining us to remove his hosiery because he wanted the carer to reapply it, and they only come on a Monday. We advised Archie that we could reapply the stockings after measuring, and we've had plenty of practice applying compression garments, but Archie still rejected our suggestion. He obviously has more trust in the donning from a carer he's known for a few months, as opposed to the professionals who order and get training on the blinking things! And he's stubborn as hell. I guess this is one of the very few aspects of his life that he can have total control over.

I then asked the TVN whether diuretics could help reduce the chronic lymphedema before a new set of stronger compression stockings was measured. The TVN said "no" to this consideration, stating that although diuretics can drain excess fluid from the body through the kidneys and improve the blood flow in the leg vessels for patients with chronic insufficiency, this medication has minimal effect on this type of swelling. Introducing it to Archie can lead to a risk of drying out other parts of the body, rather than the lymphedema and can be detrimental to Archie's general health. Archie said he would've refused to go down this route anyway, saying that it'll make him want to use the toilet more regularly, resulting in a need to increase his mobility, which will heighten the likelihood of falls at home.

Moreover, being on diuretics may lead to him not getting to the toilet in time and potentially experiencing incontinence issues. That may have created the dilemma for a short-term urethral catheter inserted to manage urine output in conjunction with the diuretic treatment. It would be an unwelcome avenue for me to have the first unfathomable experience of catheterising a bariatric patient sitting upright whilst rummaging around underneath their large apron belly. Also, from a healthcare professional's standpoint, there would be a concern that catheterisation has an infection risk and can weaken the bladder. Scarlett then piped up with her bizarre medical knowledge. She stated that if Archie got admitted to the hospital for a catheterisation, they could also consider draining his legs while they were at it. We ignored what she said, and Scarlett underestimated the role of community nurses and how Archie's condition could be adequately managed at home.

Tuesday, 4th May 2021

Today, I strongly advised Archie about the importance of leg elevation to be beneficial for lymphatic drainage. Yet, Archie explained he couldn't do this to an effective level due to the poor function of the chair. There's a concern that the existing recliner chair is no longer fit for purpose.

After the visit, I referred Archie to the occupational therapists to assess his chair and seating and examine how safe the transfers were. Archie is entirely reliant on using the recliner chair for sitting and sleeping in, and it's a medical need to alleviate leg swelling with the recliner feature of the leg rest, emphasising the necessity of doing this review. In the worst-case scenario, Archie and his wife would be willing to pay privately for a new suitable recliner chair, needing integral pressure relief and battery storage in case of power cuts. This had happened before with Archie's legs in a prolonged and sorely elevated position with cramping pains, leading to another call out for an ambulance crew to drag him out of the chair. The couple had paid for the existing recliner chair, costing £4,000 at the time; however, due to the patient's comorbidities, I wondered if Archie would be eligible for a funding scheme to help pay for a new, more appropriate chair.

Monday, 31st May 2021

We arranged a further appointment today with me, the lymphedema specialist and the TVN who visited last time. We made sure this time that Archie approved having his stockings taken off. Archie knew his carer would arrive after we left today to reapply the hosiery because three competent professionals weren't quite good enough for that task.

Archie and Scarlett were in a more pleasant mood today. Much of this was due to Archie having a brand spanking new recliner chair offered to him, thanks to the funding from the Independence at Home charity, following a grant application from the occupational therapy service after their assessment with Archie last week. Archie expects this delivery to be on Wednesday, adding, "I'll still keep hold of this one and use it as a garden chair for the summer." I don't think they've considered the logistics of how they'll keep the material dry on rainy days and how Scarlett will operate around the faulty chair and peg clothes on the washing line within their five-metre square patio. I didn't feel the need to bring this up and potentially rock the boat when we managed to get Archie to comply with our compromised plan with him.

While Archie stood out of his current chair, the lymphedema nurse so smoothly got around the legs with her measuring tape and jotted down the circumference numbers without a second thought. This is probably because the clinician had been doing more measurements for lymphedema garments than I've had hot dinners.

The completed measuring form will then have a written prescription detailing to the manufacturers the authenticity of the shape and sizes from closed toe to mid-thigh level. The garments will be a stronger class of compression this time, which will be more effective in maintaining the shaping of the lower limbs. This will prevent a multitude of consequences:

- Leg ulcers and wound infections
- Declining mobility with a high risk of a fall
- Frequent nurse visits for wound care
- Adding to the financial strain on the NHS

In the future plan, Archie agreed to continue wearing his mild compression stockings for another couple of weeks until his firmer made-to-measure hosiery arrives. If the new stockings pass the fit test once manufactured and delivered, this will be carried into Archie's long-term plan. He'll then be on the back burner of our caseload and only contacted every six months to check how he's coping with his customised garments, and if all is well with no new problems or leg pains, we can order another couple of pairs of the same stockings.

CHAPTER 6
IT'S NOT JUST A SORE FOOT

Stage one of treatment in the community (Monday, 19th April – Monday, 3rd May 2021):

A lady of 66 is living in squalor with her brother, who seems even more neglectful than her. Bianca's ghostly appearance greets you through the door, wrapped in a grey parka jacket. Her little pale face was hidden by the fluffy hood covering up to mid-eye level. Usually, the brother locks himself in his room when we come, and he's never said hello to our team. The whole interior of the house was unkempt, with dirt, cigarettes, and various forms of clutter in every room. There was no place to put my wound bag as every tabletop and floorboard had darkish brown stains, looking like a mixture of mould and cigarette ash. The smell of the place didn't have any potency through the face mask; a welcome surprise given the hideous sights from within the house.

We're seeing Bianca for twice-weekly treatments for her diabetic foot ulcer on the right heel, which developed from pressure damage during a recent hospital stay. Diabetic foot ulcers need to be acted on fast, and a referral to the diabetic foot clinic was swiftly completed. This is because 85% of patients with diabetic foot ulcers have ended up with amputations. Having a specialist team to review these wounds is important because they're at high risk of developing tissue necrosis, and the deterioration of these wounds isn't helped by the common feature of diabetics, which is their lack of sensation in their feet. A sensory neuropathy test using a 10-gram monofilament pen is a good indicator for measuring the blood flow in the feet, which we also tested with Bianca initially in her care. It can be beneficial to try the monofilament pen on the patient's wrist first to reassure them that it'll feel like a feather rather than poking them with a needle, especially if they're needle phobic. There are 10 sites on each foot to touch with the monofilament pen while their eyes are closed, and they tell me when they feel a point in their foot being pressed. If they feel eight sites or less, this will indicate a loss of protective sensation. In Bianca's case, she scored a 5/10 for sensation on both feet and, therefore, is affected by diabetic neuropathy.

Suppose a person with diabetes gets an infection in an undiagnosed foot wound. Unfortunately, this can lead to gangrene, affecting cell, skin, and tissue death and loss, resulting in amputations of feet and limbs, which may become non-functional pieces of rotten flesh and are no good to man or beast. Surprisingly and frustratingly (on top of all the other poor hospital discharges lately), Bianca was just advised to treat this open category three pressure ulcer with E45 cream (not even a first-choice emollient cream for us). One might ask, "Did we prescribe this lady a course of antibiotics because her wound was smelly, painful and with lobster-red surrounding skin?" To them, I'll say, "Yes, you're right, Sherlock Holmes." Having the moist wound exposed without a dressing and living in a grotty household would probably have been the critical factors for the obvious wound infection. The laboratory later confirmed from our wound swab that it was positive for staphylococcus aureus, the primary hardy pathogen typically found in infected wounds in the community, as it can be easily spread in the household. We need to be wary, as this pathogen can develop a resistance to antibiotics known as MRSA. This growing epidemic is why we wash our hands or use alcohol-based sanitiser before and after patient contact. PPE is to be worn for clinical procedures with infection risks, and the aseptic non-touch technique will be used. MRSA cannot be taken lightly for any visits or families living with the service users of our concern, and they should also frequently wash their hands and wash their clothes, towels, and bed linen to avoid the spread of this super-bug because it has the capability of causing severe infections, leading to sepsis and death.

A diabetic foot wound may not reveal the typical signs of a wound infection. Bianca's wound didn't because there wasn't heat felt or erythema seen on the intact surrounding skin. One useful observation you can do in this situation is to check the patient's blood sugar levels. When we did this for Bianca, her recordings were in the mid to high teens. We didn't think the inadequate dietary intake of occasional peanut butter and jam sandwiches would trigger the higher-than-average readings. I knew that a wound infection could elevate blood sugar levels, and this is what I clinically suspected.

We initially had to ponder about the correct type of dressing to put on the far-from-healthy-looking wound. The cost of managing wounds in the NHS across the UK was claimed to be £8.3 billion in 2017/18, though according to Public Policy Projects, this is believed to have risen to £10 billion a year, which are common comorbidities for the patients I see on my caseload. In addition to this, two-thirds of the costs in community nursing settings are spent on wound care. With these statistics in mind, and what I already brought to the readers' attention in my previous memoir, wound care is a heavy financial burden on the NHS. This is one of the reasons why practitioners dealing with wounds need to make cost-effective decisions, as well as healing the wound up as quickly as possible without further health deficits to the patients in question.

We decided to commence an iodine-putty dressing in our wound care regime, not only to offer an antimicrobial covering but to attach itself to the wound bed and debride away the nasty, slimy, sloughy tissue. Slough isn't what we want to see on a wound bed, and it's the initial feature of devitalised tissue in the wound and is a yellow colour. We want to remove the slough to see the granulation tissue, which we may find straight away from an injury with partial thickness skin loss. After seeing slough, we want to start seeing granulation tissue in the worse-looking wound beds, as it indicates the remodelling phase of the skin structure.

The toenails on Bianca's feet didn't help matters. They were all long and thickened with a dark yellow discoloured appearance, and Bianca couldn't remember when they were last trimmed and filed back. Therefore, completing an urgent referral to the podiatry service was added to my to-do list. Having the toenails professionally cut and filed back will help preclude an injury to her toes. If a patient is showing signs of fungal infection in their thickened toenails and if they have undiagnosed athlete's foot, then this can spread up to the foot and leg, preventing any ulcers from healing.

In a past wound care conference I attended, it was said that the average person walks around the earth five times in a lifetime. We, therefore, must take care of our feet because they've done so much for us to get through life. One way of doing this is choosing the correct footwear, which will decrease the risks of pressure sores developing in the heels and toes, a pronounced bunion on the edge of the great toes, or even the fluid-filled swelling of a ganglion near the ankle joint, which may affect a cluster of nerve cells. For Bianca, in the initial phase of her care, we recommend that she use a pair of pressure-relieving shoes. With her blessing, we measured her feet and took from our nursing store cupboard a pair of black therapeutic shoes manufactured with an 18-millimetre thick multi-foam insole. We detached small removable blocks at the plantar area of the insole to design an offloading function for her vulnerable heels. Another benefit to this footwear is its inclusion of fastening Velcro straps to prevent the shoes from slipping off the foot when taking steps and having this extra feature reduces the possibility of falls, which, as I've already discovered, is a high risk of occurring for my patients who are above the age of 65. We emphasised that these specialised shoes should be used simply for standing and walking and taken off when Bianca is offloading her heels using a footstool or lying on her grubby settee to sleep.

Stage two of treatment (Monday, 3rd May – Monday, 17th May 2021):

Before one of the visits, our nurse, Rachel, contacted Bianca's mobile, but there was no answer on two occasions. It later transpired that Bianca dislikes speaking on the phone because it makes her feel nervous. Even though Bianca is mobile enough to get out of the house, she can't attend the local GP practice regularly or a clinic appointment. This is due to her crippling anxiety, which is the main reason for the referral to the community nurses. It also became troubling to us that there might be an imbalance of dependence or power between Bianca and her brother in the home. As Rachel was the same nurse going into the house for continuity, Bianca was able to be more open about her life.

Bianca is sleeping on her brother's sofa and can't wait to have her own space and company again. Rachel asked Bianca where she'd like to relocate if she could leave her brother's address. In response, Bianca said she wanted to move to a bungalow (council-owned), which her social worker from Devon had worked hard to arrange for her. This new home for her will be just outside our geographical attachment area. Thus, she'll be under a different GP practice and community nursing service. Bianca explained it was ready for her to move into it, having been newly refurbished, and she'd bought a £700 Persian rug and got it delivered to the bungalow. Her nephew would put up curtain rails, which was the final task that needed doing. She was frustrated that she hadn't yet seen this place, let alone live there.

Bianca went on to say that even though she's ready to move on, there's a fear that her brother won't be able to cope financially with his care and independent living. Bianca said that he suffers from back pain and stays in bed most of the time, not always taking his medication and only eating bananas and digestive biscuits. She gets him drinks of water and makes him cups of tea, which he demands to be made a certain way; milk, then teabag, then hot water.

"And he can tell if it's done wrong," Bianca adds. "I've tested it before, and he doesn't miss a trick regarding tea making." Bianca goes on to say that she pays for her brother's bills and pays for their combined food shop, which another relative physically gets and delivers to the house. She also bought a brand-new washing machine last week, and at present, she doesn't have a bank card because she gave it to her brother and niece to go shopping, and they lost her card on that trip. She contacted her bank and cancelled the card when she realised she hadn't yet received a new one. Bianca said it was lucky she kept a hidden wad of cash in the house for safekeeping.

When Rachel then mentioned the predicament about the brother and whether he'd contemplate having care set up and not relying on her, Bianca replied that he's incredibly stubborn and won't accept help. Bianca has an open referral to the mental health team due to her depression and anxiety. She speaks highly of her case holder from Devon, with whom she has stayed in touch since they met. Bianca told Rachel that she'd also been in touch with a lady from the Red Cross charity when she was last in hospital. Although she didn't want to talk to anybody from the Red Cross until she moved into the new bungalow, she was still happy for the community nurses to contact social services to support her with moving into the bungalow and discuss the brother's financial dependence on her.

In the handover, Rachel said how nervous Bianca appeared when the brother was brought into the conversation. She lowered her voice to almost a whisper, saying her brother was probably listening from the room next door. With that, Rachel unmuted the television and turned it up slightly, allowing Bianca to speak more freely. It was troubling to Rachel that Bianca felt uneasy about her brother overhearing things and that he had a bad temper. We approached the subsequent visits to seek further investigations and conversed all concerns with Adult Services, including the recent hints of financial abuse.

On the next visit, Bianca wanted to talk about her brother again, but she wanted to do this discreetly. So, Rachel closed the door between the living room and the hallway that leads to the brother's bedroom, and she and Rachel spoke in hushed tones. Bianca repeatedly said she wanted to leave her brother's home and move into the new bungalow. Rachel told Bianca that this had been discussed with social services following our current referral, and somebody from their team would visit to assist her with the desperate move. Time was of the essence, and I was perturbed that she may otherwise lose the tenancy for the property.

Bianca said her brother got stuck on the toilet last night, and a neighbour got called in to help heave out his saggy bottom away from the toilet bowl that formed a suction seal inside the rim. It is an unfortunate moment that everyone other than the brother can reflect on with a smirk. He then told Bianca to ask Rachel to order a raised toilet seat. As we cannot prescribe NHS equipment for parties other than the patient, Rachel wrote a note for the brother to contact the GP and request a referral to occupational therapy.

Rachel felt apprehension for the brother and asked Bianca if they could stick their head into the bedroom and check if he was OK, but Bianca immediately shook her head and muttered, "He's disgusting. All he does is lie in bed and eat bananas and biscuits." Bianca elaborated by saying that he'd left his niece's French bulldog food in a bowl on the kitchen counter all night for when the niece came over with them in the morning, "which was also disgusting, too," she added. Rachel didn't want to press further to check on the brother as they knew it would cause Bianca to be upset, and they were concerned it might break her trust in him.

On the update regarding the pressure wound on the heel, the flucloxacillin that the GP lengthened to a two-week course knocked back the infection signs, and the red erythema, heat and soreness subsided. It continues to show a circular necrotic plug, which needs debriding. Necrotic tissue isn't good to see on a wound and is usually seen as dark, firm, devitalised tissue but can also become soft and boggy. To debride the necrosis, we apply thin, small slabs of honey dressings over the top to moisten and eventually lift the devitalised tissue. We also cover the honey with an absorbent pad and bandage Bianca from toe to knee because otherwise, the honey will stick like shit to a blanket. In this case, it'll be a filthy, grubby floor and furniture with a whole spectrum of nasty pathogens lurking around and wanting to immigrate on the heel wound with moist living conditions for them to thrive.

Stage three of treatment (Monday, 17th May – Thursday, 10th June 2021):

It then became my turn to visit, and I also ended up having an interesting conversation, learning more about this lady's life while kneeling on the floor of the squalid living room doing wound care on the heel. She spoke at length about her past. Bianca said she had a promising start in life, working alongside her former husband, a successful self-employed tree surgeon, so much so that their carving creations were auctioned to public parks and schools nationwide. A large tree trunk remaining vertical was carved into a giant squirrel. Another chunk of an oak tree was sculptured horizontally into a crocodile. Both wooden creatures are used for the outdoor entertainment of children. They are brilliant additions to the playground facilities and made a morning TV show at one point for the public to feast their eyes on the craftsmanship belonging to this marvellous creator. This led to them buying their own three-bedroom house in their mid-twenties, much to the distaste of her bitter brother, who has always had a bit of a domestic rivalry.

Bianca was living her best life of wealth, success, and fortune. So where did it go wrong for this dishevelled-looking woman I see before me? Dominic then spoke briefly about a marriage breakdown with her ex-husband later in her life. "He had it off with my best friend at the time... and she was the bridesmaid at my wedding..." Bianca gazed glumly at the floor, and I changed the subject of conversation after that statement to avoid sparking another depressive episode. I then brought up about the ongoing safeguarding issues. After suspicions of financial abuse from the brother and niece, Bianca still hasn't received her new bank card in the post following the closure of her previous card. Bianca then elaborated on the current situation with her brother, saying that he's a fire hazard because he constantly smokes cigarettes in his room, and she's seen him fall asleep in bed with a cigarette still in his mouth. Bianca also expressed her concern about her brother's deterioration in health. Bianca noticed that his ankles have become very swollen because he stays in his room all day and has been known to even defecate and urinate in the bedroom. She said that her brother refuses any care or health checks; this message was relayed to the nursing team after the visit.

Bianca is none the wiser about knowing when to move into her new property. In a conversation with the GP earlier in the day, they informed me that they'd get in touch with Bianca's social worker and caseworker from Devon, as both had been heavily involved in securing the bungalow. The doctor also addressed that whilst Bianca was living in her previous flat, she'd been battling with alcohol abuse, and the brother had apparently helped her a lot during that time. Since Bianca's latest hospital discharge (she was admitted after a fall with a long lie and a background of alcohol excess), the doctor believes that Bianca has been sober in recent weeks, and the nurses, including Rachel and myself, haven't seen any alcohol near her possession in the visits. Maybe having a sobering state could explain why Bianca has new insight and why a new narrative about the relationship with her brother has surfaced.

Later that week, the niece received a phone call from the physical disabilities social worker who completed an in-person assessment of Bianca at her brother's home with a view of taking her to the new bungalow. Going forward, the social worker will also support Bianca with her bank account and make sure her missing bank card is sent to the new address, setting up a lifeline, organising a referral to occupational therapy, organising a package of care if it becomes appropriate (Bianca has declined this in the past), and keeping an eye on the potential dependence her brother had been displaying whilst she lived with him. Social services will also contact Bianca's brother at a future date to offer a care-needs assessment for him as it seems apparent that he's struggling with his own care needs, and although Bianca has had to stay at her brother's to look after the niece's docile dog, the care for the pet will now need complete management from the niece unless Bianca will be open to more dog-sitting to keep her company.

A further update on the pressure ulcer on the heel: much of the dark necrotic plug had lifted off. Our nursing team continued using honey dressings underneath an absorbent pad and soft bandaging to remove the remaining slough at the base of the wound until it showed full granulation tissue. Bianca has remained compliant with our advice, wearing her pressure-relieving shoes in the daytime unless she's offloading her heels by a different means, as stated in the initial phase of treatment.

It was fortunate for Bianca to be referred to our team to get this ball successfully rolling in the first place, and as well as that, we're improving her heel wound, which is becoming smaller and drier, and wound care has been reduced to weekly visits. She'll hopefully attend her appointment with the diabetic foot clinic next week, which can review and make extra alterations to the wound care regime. It's reasonable to say that Bianca's relatively short time under the nursing service has turned into a success story that we all hope will progress into a more stabilised life for her. We're very grateful to social services and the physical disabilities team, as much of this success goes towards their intervention.

Monday, 21st June 2021

The following week, Bianca's brother was admitted to the hospital by the paramedics, having turned down any medical or social support, resulting in his crisis point where he was found slumped forward on the bed and unable to sit up straight, being a risk of suffocation in the duvet. On a promising note, the brother's house looks almost immaculate, having been deep cleaned by the family all week. Once more, Bianca now has her bank card replacement with access to her savings, thanks to the help of his social worker.

CHAPTER 7
THE COMPLEXITIES OF PHYSICAL AND MENTAL HEALTH ISSUES

Tucked away from a main road and amongst the overgrown trees and bushes lies a dilapidated cottage. Inside this cottage lives Merlin, an 80-year-old, and his medical history includes stable heart failure, COPD, generalised osteoarthritis, depressive episodes, split personality disorder, and long-term lymphedema for 30 years. With all these comorbidities comes a long list of medications. He had his medications stored in Dossette boxes, which are in a pile on a dinner table on the opposite side of the room, and they're dispensed routinely by the carers. Dossette boxes are ideal for a complicated medication regime, like Merlin's, with various pills taken at different times of the day. The tablets are in small plastic compartments that clearly label which medicines must be given at what time of day.

Besides Merlin's medication regime, though, the presenting problems of this gentleman were bilateral oedematous legs, which are leaking. The skin on the legs felt firm and lumpy with papillomatosis, resembling a pebble-dash wall design painted in a beige colour with tinges of red. It is a feature from congestion of the blood circulation due to uncontrolled lymphedema. Prominent patches of hyperkeratosis were also built up on the legs, which resembled thick, dark tree bark. An abnormality where the skin produces extra layers of keratin for protection from excessive pressure, inflammation and irritation to the skin. These features are despite continuous cycles of community nursing treatment.

For most people, walking is an ability that's not only essential in everyday life but is also something that's entirely taken for granted when you can do it so effortlessly. Since working around people who are physically disabled and those who have reduced mobility through age and life-threatening and debilitating conditions (which Merlin is in the bracket of) I've come to appreciate walking as another blessing in my life because it offers so much to one's life. Walking can be used for exercise, and with that comes improved health and enjoyment purposes. Walking also gives an individual independence in numerous ways, and a better quality of life comes with all these positive aspects.

With many of the service users I visit, their quality of life is already impacted because they have poor mobility and will therefore be disadvantaged in achieving the benefits stated above, the main one being independence. When mobility becomes so limited, there are biomechanical issues with the body due to postural difficulties from sitting in an awkward position in an inappropriate, non-comforting chair for too long and muscle wastage in the legs, which affect how long you can weight bear your whole body in a standing position. One of the biggest problems I see with my armchair patients is their reduced ankle range of motion. The ankle is classed as the machine that operates the foot and calf muscle pump; the second most important muscle for pumping blood around the body, other than the heart muscle. When there's a decreased ankle range of motion, this will be the main contributing factor to venous insufficiency, occurring when your leg veins don't allow blood to flow back up to heart level. The condition leads to swollen legs with varicose veins and the development of leg ulcers. It's also a big contributor to the dysfunction of the lymphatic system, leading to the challenging, chronic condition of lymphedema. Lymphedema builds up and worsens when the balance is disturbed between the fluid exchange from the blood capillaries in the veins and an imbalance of what's drained from the lymphatic system, which is too minuscule to see but runs along the veins. The more severe the chronic oedema is, the higher the chance of skin tissue becoming hardened with the build-up of hyperkeratosis and papillomatosis becoming evident, and Merlin is undoubtedly at that stage. What's extra concerning (as noted in a wound care conference) is that it increases the risk of deep vein thrombosis and heart failure.

The formidable challenge with Merlin was that he's chairfast due to pains in the arthritic joints of his legs and does NOT elevate his legs, not even overnight, regardless of us nagging him about this, like a frustrating mother at a disobedient child for not doing their homework. On the topic of pain, it's described by the National Institute for Health and Care Excellence (NICE) as being chronic when it lasts more than three months. The term' chronic pain' – sometimes recognised as long-term or persistent pain – can refer to various painful disorders. It can be secondary to underlying osteoarthritis, rheumatoid arthritis, ulcerative colitis, or endometriosis. Chronic pain can also be the primary injury, with no precise diagnosis, or the pain (or its effect) appears to be out of proportion to any observable injury or condition. NICE claimed in 2021 that chronic pain affected an estimated one-third to one-half of the UK's population.

Despite chronic pain being a common complaint in healthcare, patients are still poorly managed, having their quality of life impacted, and the British Pain Society identified depression and loss of employment as major consequences. On top of this, Merlin's also very stubborn in his behaviour and will NOT go to bed upstairs. He also will NOT allow certain staff members to visit him.

The Complexities of Physical and Mental Health Issues

He has his favourite nurses, which he's entitled to have, but he makes it known to all staff members, and he has tendencies to play one staff member off over another. "Can you not send Nurse X to see me again, please? She's too strict with me, and I don't like the way they put the bandaging on my legs. It's too tight. Just add her to my naughty list, would you?" When he said this to me, I replied, "You can't pick and choose who can come and visit you, Merlin, because we don't always have the staff levels and skill mixes to accommodate patient preferences. But I'll report your concerns to the office, and we'll see what we can do."

Merlin gets easily emotional with low moods. He gets triggered with negative emotions when you bring up his family; thus, it's difficult to maintain pleasant conversations in the house when you're knelt opposite him, spending at least an hour per visit providing the treatments. He'll say how much he misses his former wife, and he always misses his daughter, who still sees Merlin regularly despite working full-time as a chef in a local restaurant and looking after her disabled son as a single parent. Patients displaying signs of anxiety and depression should always be carefully monitored under our care, especially when the patient presents with wounds, because multiple studies have shown that anxiety and depression impair the healing process. Low moods have been known to slow wound healing due to the interference of the hormone cortisol, which affects the production of anti-inflammatory substances called cytokines, causing a wound to remain sore and inflamed for longer.

Merlin has infinite scratch marks and wounds around his body. They scab up and reopen due to Merlin constantly scratching himself. He says he has an undiagnosed skin condition, yet my team associates the scratching with his psychological status. We're basing this on experiencing his often unstable emotions on visits and knowing about his countless readmissions to mental institutes for rehab and his extensive medical background of anxiety, depression and being known to the mental health services. I also suspect that the scratching started as a psychological problem; a form of self-abuse. Over time, I imagine that the skin has become irritable, developing similar traits to his own, and the itchiness from the scratch wounds drying and scabbing up causes Merlin more of an urge to scratch until they bleed. It's not just the legs that are affected by this psychological issue. An endless number of minor rounded, scabbed wounds around the neck, shoulder blades, lower back, buttocks, tummy and thighs cover the skin like tattoos. The fact that he's had no ambition to do anything other than to watch the television, eat and manoeuvre his wide load to the commode beside him in an awkward fashion must send him to extreme boredom. Adding to his depression and reliance on social contact when he's had enough hours of sleep in her system and a chirpier mood. I've wondered whether the fear of losing our service is another motive for all this self-abusing, as that would mean fewer people to talk to twice weekly.

Blood stains are completely encased into the carpet below him, all around the front of his ragged brown chair, which they refuse to give up and replace, even though Merlin knows he can get funding for a more modern, bespoke, state-of-the-art chair due to fitting the eligibility for hospital avoidance. These blood stains from his scratched wounds that come and go are an added reminder of the many years of self-abuse and neglect. Rolls of tissues are on either side of the chair, nestled in the clutter with the crisps, sweet treats, and cans of fizzy drinks, which he thought we couldn't see on his cupboard shelves. When tempted to have another good scratch, the bog roll is squeezed inside her rucked-up bandaging to control further bleeding.

The helpful information we gathered from Merlin came from a discharge summary a decade ago. According to the summary, Merlin was admitted with alarmingly swollen legs with cellulitis and had papillomatosis, like the initial presentation under the community nurses. Once the cellulitis was treated with antibiotics, Merlin's legs were dried up and healed. Skin became smooth with a much better leg shape, and this was due to Merlin being in compression bandaging and having his legs elevated in bed. For that reason, we went forward with the subsequent phases of treatment, having that knowledge in our arsenal.

Stage one of treatment in the community (Monday, 4th January – Monday, 18th January 2021):

There was no record of a Doppler apart from input from the vascular service a couple of years ago, who determined that strong compression would be suitable for Merlin's legs. We were unable to determine accurate readings from a Doppler assessment, yet in conjunction with the previous story of Archie, a joint visit with a TVN for an evaluation based on clinical judgment was undertaken instead. In this examination, we could identify normal temperature in the legs, good capillary refill in the toes and no peripheral neuropathy in the feet. Based on the clinical assessment, we trialled, with caution, strong compression bandaging on one leg whilst carrying on with mild compression bandaging on the other leg for one week. It turned out that the more robust compression led to no adverse effects on the leg, so it became the treatment for bilateral legs.

Stage two of treatment (Monday, 18th January – Monday, 15th February 2021):

Merlin wasn't managing with bandaging when visits were once a week as he had tendencies to push down the bandaging so he could scratch his skin, which was itchy as well as sore. It was also challenging for us nurses to apply the bandaging due to Merlin's osteoarthritis. When lifting his right leg, it would sound like the rickety wooden floorboards of a rusty old ship, and you can tell from the forlorn face Merlin was pulling and the recurrent groaning noises that it's been increasingly uncomfortable for him to receive treatment over time. It makes it very hard to operate the wound care, especially around the back of the legs, where the skin is only a couple of inches away from the chair. It's also strenuous to apply the compression bandaging at the correct degree of tension when the rotund legs are naturally clumped together with little space to separate them and do our thing with the gold-standard level of care.

Visits were then increased to three times a week, and we provided bowl washes each time with an emollient to aid debridement of hyperkeratosis. Under TVN guidance, we also initiated a two-week trial of a paste bandage soaked in zinc oxide and ichthammol, which are ingredients to help soothe the skin and ease any itching and irritation.

Stage three of treatment (Monday, 15th February – Monday, 8th March 2021):

Over one month, things improved for Merlin. The leg shape normalised, skin became drier, and her knobbly papillomatosis disappeared. This still didn't diminish how the legs were still abnormally shaped for the standard compression stockings you can order from the catalogue, and they needed to be measured for made-to-measure hosiery instead at a thigh-length where the non-shifting oedema was lurking.

My team didn't think Merlin's legs would reduce any further in size unless he elevated his legs. We tried negotiating with Merlin to use his bed upstairs, even if it was just for afternoon bedrests, but this idea backfired. When this was discussed, Merlin refused to go upstairs again, let alone use the bed. It was a decision Merlin made when his wife passed away several years ago. He still has the same double bed, which they shared, and he doesn't want to see it as it'll upset him as it'll be a reminder of a loving marriage that abruptly got taken away from him through a ferocious form of cancer. Merlin doesn't want to remove the bed from his house either because it makes it feel like he still has part of her with him. Indeed, there are other solutions to using a bed, I hear you ask. Well, unfortunately, not. Merlin doesn't want to have a bed downstairs because he doesn't want to deal with the decluttering, and it appears he wants to remain a hoarder. Living within his squalor with plenty of garbage that he wouldn't even realise exists. You cannot win over certain things with patients and their stubbornness.

By this point, there became less of a need for the paste bandaging and to maintain the prevention of skin irritation, but there were still exacerbations of Merlin's skin picking disorder, even though he denied the accusations of scratching his legs. When we noticed this, we applied short-term courses of Diprosalic ointment to the skin, the same topical steroid cream that's helped clear away hyperkeratosis for others under the TVN guidance.

Stage four with treatment (Monday, 8th March – Wednesday, 4th August 2021):

The fit-testing of the customised compression stockings was successful, and the skincare regime and management of the hosiery were under the shared care of Merlin's care agency. A comprehensive care plan was written and emailed to the agency for education on our shared care advice. This lasted five months without a visit from a community nurse; however, exacerbations of skin irritation, ripping skin to shreds with scratching and weeping bloody exudate from the damaged skin, happened too frequently. Merlin ultimately required further face-to-face appointments for community nursing treatment.

Repeated spells of being unwell due to exacerbations of COPD, recurrent urinary tract infections and chest infections didn't help with a setback like this. These medical issues usually occur at least every month, adding to the vicious cycle of negative emotions endured and heightening the risk of Merlin's skin integrity deterioration on the body map. Merlin's daughter going away on holiday with her son for two weeks was also problematic for him at this point. When visiting Merlin, he explained how attached he was to his daughter and dependent on her for support and to arrive with his favourite Victoria sponge cake that she'd occasionally whip up for him in her kitchen. Merlin feared that his daughter would abandon him because he felt that he'd been a bad father and that she didn't want to deal with his grief.

The fifth and final stage of treatment in the community (Wednesday, 4th August 2021, until further notice):

Things perked up again for Merlin once his daughter returned from her holiday and when we stopped 'hassling' him to make changes in their daily routine (for his own good). A vascular assessment based on clinical judgement was conducted again, and similar readings were gathered. As before, equal treatment was followed with the paste bandage and the strong compression bandaging.

Merlin's leg condition drastically improved again after several weeks. Then it was recommended by a TVN to re-measure the legs and thighs for customised stockings, but with a stronger class of compression to avoid any rebound oedema or problematic flareups, and without the silicone banding at the top of the thighs as this led to more itching. Knowing that the carers would struggle with the donning and doffing of firmer hosiery, we also ordered a stocking applicator for them to use. When this all came into play, Merlin's chronic lymphedema was managed well under long-term shared care. On occasions, though, the carers have been given additional telephone advice. For example, whether to re-start topical steroid treatment if flareups of excoriated skin occurred.

In a review of the outcome of this episode of care, it ended up being a success story for a very complex patient with multiple challenges. Continuity of care was vital. Our clinical judgement determined the suitability for strong compression, which was a game changer. Merlin noticed improvements, and this uplifted his mood, which also assisted with healing his leg ulcers. Humour proved to help with Merlin's compliance in wearing his hosiery, too. Merlin noticed that his name was sown into the tags of his stockings – obviously how the manufacturing company do things for each client, and I joked with Merlin that he could have his own brand of compression garments called "Merlin's sexy legs." Keeping the carers on our side with shared care has also been crucial in maintaining our success. By that, I mean providing individualised care plans and being available to listen to concerns and offer advice as and when necessary.

CHAPTER 8
EVERY SERVICE HAS ITS FAULTS

Friday, 3rd September 2021

I finished my shift a lot later than planned, no thanks to zero help tonight when I should have been assigned another nurse and health care assistant. What's worse is that I suspected that the catheter inserted for that lady I just visited wasn't even in the right place to start with. I always get some urine flowing from a service user I successfully catheterise, irrespective of who they are. Yet, there was zero urine in the night bag, and instead, the urine bypassed the tubing and soaked the bedsheets. And when I went in with a fresh, sterile catheter into the bladder, it drained 500 millilitres immediately. The main purpose for attending the patient's address in the first place (as instructed by the daytime triage nurse) was for bowel care, but it was obvious in the end that this lady wasn't constipated. I visited well beyond the daytime shift because the GP had a long delay in prescribing the four-gram glycerine suppositories. Then, the husband had to collect it from the pharmacy before I could start the 'essential' interventions.

Glycerine suppositories encourage the bowels to empty stools in mild to moderate constipation. If laxative suppositories or mini enemas don't aid bowel movement, then a phosphate enema should be a last resort, but they're never to be administered by district nurses. Too much rectal sodium phosphate may cause serious kidney or heart damage and can lead to death, especially for someone as vulnerable as this lady.

When I did a rectal examination on the patient, they didn't feel compacted with faeces, but I feared there may've been higher compaction in the bowels. I decided to administer the suppository, and when I did this, the husband piped up and commented that his wife had opened her bowels daily for the last four days by doing the manual evacuation himself. He said he used to work in care, and the nurse practitioner from the surgery was happy with him continuing the bowel care after guiding him through it on the first day. I doubt that's what the husband thought he had in store when he said "through sickness and in health" in the wedding vows.

Regardless of his wife's regular bowel motion, he watched me proceed with unnecessary bowel care because he still thought she was bunged up at the start of the visit. But to cut a long story short, everything that happened to this lady today, before my encounter, was completely inappropriate. I informed my line manager on WhatsApp right away when I got home, who said she'd escalate the issues I've raised in the band seven meeting, which was fittingly tomorrow. She agreed that it appeared to be a failed triage from the outset this morning, which is unacceptable and meant that I went into overtime hours yet again, not helped by the extra hour driving to the patient's postcode at the furthest point away from my base. I also decided to send my full reflection on tonight's shift to our Head of Nursing to address the problems and that our current out-of-hour service is not efficient enough. Hopefully, things get ironed out from the feedback.

It's been the first week of this new late system, where my shift is meant to finish at 8 p.m. when the private night nurse service takes over for the next 12 hours until the daytime service starts again. Today demonstrated how much we rely on at least two nurses covering all geographical areas during the out-of-hours times, and it would've saved me the long journey over.

Friday, 24th September 2021

You know you're among healthcare workers when you discuss puke and bowel movements at the lunch table, and no one flinches. From a nurse's perspective, sometimes you may get carried away with this fact in your personal life. Today, I was sitting at the dinner table with my girlfriend and her dad at their home, and it got onto the subject of work. I spoke about a recently challenging visit I cannot get out of my head. In detail, I talk about a failed catheter insertion with a male patient, known for being difficult in the past with painful catheterisations. In one procedure, he needed gas and air in the hospital.

Although my failed catheter insertion caused a degree of pain for this poor gentleman, despite using the anaesthetic lubrication gel, that wasn't the only thing I was bothered by on the visit. My main concern was scraping his prostate on every failed attempt, even though I got him to cough, which has been a useful tip for male catheter users in widening the passageway from the urethra to the bladder.

Unfortunately, on this recent visit, there were clear signs of dark haematuria in the top of the catheter tubing to signal that I was causing internal damage, likely to the prostate, based on the resistance I was getting at a premature level. This led to an admission to A&E, which is never a swift, straightforward process at the best of times, especially not on a Friday afternoon. The 89-year-old gentleman didn't help matters as he didn't want to be picked up by an ambulance or a care car because he didn't want to pay for a taxi back home, and I was advised that he didn't drive himself in case he exacerbated the abdominal pain or the bleed from his penis. He's due a driving test next week to check whether he can retain his driver's licence because his eyesight is worsening. Rather than driving to the hospital, the patient wore an incontinence pad underneath his trousers, and he waited for his less-than-impressed son to travel 30 miles to pick up his dad.

After I told this story, my girlfriend's dad said he didn't want to hear gruesome nursing stories from me anymore. Including when it involves blood and we're eating a beetroot curry. Sometimes, I must remind myself around my non-medical friends not to talk about problems with patients and their bodily functions.

Monday, 11th October 2021

Once the crisis of COVID had settled down and restrictions were reduced, the nursing office became busy once again with an array of visitors. Periodically, these would be representatives of medical products, often catheter suppliers. They were handsome salespeople in their 20s and 30s and dressed in designer clothing. They'd have so much excitement and a willingness to engage in conversation, which seemed abnormal compared to the feelings around the office from the nurses after some tough visits. But because these male reps always came with pizzas, pens, notepads and other gifts, the lady nurses made them feel welcome as soon as their presence was known. And I was equally engaging with them purely because of my hunger for pizza.

Monday, 1st November 2021

A spooky story was told at handover today regarding a service user who sadly passed away at one of our residential homes. The nurse couldn't help but notice the bewildered look on the senior carer's face when they asked if there were any details about the death. Were they in bed and asleep? Was it a comfortable death? The senior carer said that at 4:20 a.m. this morning, she happened to be there for the patient's final breath with a colleague when they were doing their four-hourly turns for the patient on the bed (as we advised in the care plan) to allow for pressure relief to all pressure areas. This information was emphasised when we noticed a deep tissue injury on the patient's spine. The senior carer then told the nurse that when they glanced at his watch, it had stopped at the exact same time as his death. The carer added with a stutter that the watch worked fine during the day because she'd used it to check his respiratory rate.

Tuesday, 23rd November 2021

"Sorry, but we don't deal with frequent fliers." This was what a healthcare assistant told a service user today when she refused to provide wound care for a skin tear on the patient's arm. The HCA had a valid point with her comment because this patient always leaves their house and is accident-prone. The patient also rushed to A&E with her daughter last month when she broke her nose, falling into the front door with her groceries.

I then searched for other stories relating to inappropriate referrals on the district nursing humour page on Facebook, and it didn't fail to amuse me. And I've experienced or heard similarities to these stories in my handovers.

One nurse wrote on a Facebook post that her patient recently said they couldn't attend the clinic, and when she rang the landline to arrange a house call, the patient had gone on the bus to go shopping in the town centre.

Another service user had once told a nurse that they were housebound but couldn't do Thursday mornings as they go to the hairdressers.

A different nurse went to administer a flu vaccine for a 'housebound' person and found him up a tree picking apples at the bottom of an exceedingly long garden.

On a separate occasion, the patient told a nurse that they couldn't drive and because they have reduced mobility now, they're deemed housebound, so they can't get to the treatment clinic. The nurse then goes into KFC a few hours later to get lunch, and lo and behold, they see the same patient in there on their own, eating a bucket of chicken with lots of shopping bags. The next day, that same nurse sent a letter through the patient's door advising them to attend the treatment room for the above reasons.

These incidents happened more so before the COVID-19 pandemic, and I feel our service has gained deserving respect in recent years. You may still get the odd, surprising request from a newbie, asking, "Could you make it early? I'm catching the train at 10." That might be because people are unaware of the role of a community nurse and what meets the criteria for seeing one before they're referred to us, usually by a nescient GP.

Other times, you get the ones that use and abuse our service. The housebound ones need timed visits so they don't have to stop in and wait. Then you turn up later than planned, and when you arrive, they have a face like thunder in their armchair and say, "Where have you been? I've been waiting all day for you!"

Friday, 17th December 2021

A HCA came into the office today after finishing her insulin round, which is her duty most days in our team at the moment. She was holding up a pair of yellow knitted gloves. She said it was given to her by the wife of one of our diabetic patients. The husband kept saying that the HCA's hands were cold in the morning when checking the blood sugar levels and giving insulin injections into his abdomen, and the wife took this matter into her own hands. Over the last month, the wife had been knitting the HCA a pair of gloves to warm up her hands during the morning rounds. The stitching was a bit out of alignment in places, but her Alzheimer's is progressing, and it's the thought that counts at Christmas, right? This is probably the sweetest thing I've heard all year.

Monday, 27th December 2021

Monday mornings can be the worst feeling at work, including when you're 10 emails down a chain and working out where you fit into the conversation between the TVNs, lymphedema specialist and a clinical rep. The typical Monday morning mood is similar for many other nurses today, the first day after boxing day. Not just because you're back to reality too quickly after some quality family time, but you may also see that people have overeaten at Christmas and haven't been to the toilet for days. You may get the joy of visiting Betty with faecal impaction and discussing the laxative pathway with them.

CHAPTER 9
TIME TO TAKE A STAND

Thursday, 24th February 2022

Today, it was announced that Russia launched a full-scale invasion of Ukraine and occupied parts of it. Millions of people have fled, and others have stayed to fight. I'm in disbelief about such dreadful news so soon after getting through a global pandemic. All our hearts from the UK go out to the people of Ukraine. I'm lost for words…

Friday, 18th March 2022

In recent times, on a 'quiet' Friday afternoon, our service suddenly enters a baptism of fire. Previously, we received a referral from a patient's carer regarding new pressure damage at three p.m. Another time, we received a referral from a patient's spouse to say that their husband's catheter had been blocked for six hours, and when we looked at the clock, it was four p.m. Other times, we get the 4:15 p.m. hospital discharges, typically for end-of-life care or poor old Bob, who's returned to the local residential home with a new sore on their bottom. You've not only got to attend the initial visit, but you must complete the endless paperwork, consisting of a progress note, devising a care plan and planning future appointments. If it's a new pressure ulcer you need to complete an incident report, detailing the cause of the injury and what pressure relieving advice has been verbally given to the caregivers.

An unexpected late referral approached us today. It got to 3:30 p.m., and the triage nurse asked me to visit patient X, who has bilateral leaky legs. When I arrived, I could see the bandaging was sodden in exudate. One of the legs had suspected signs of cellulitis, and I decided to leave this one out of the compression bandaging as it was more swollen than the other; the skin was bright red with erythema, and he had some degree of pain with it. Not only did the visit take an hour long, but I was also ringing the doctor's surgery to request antibiotics. I'm then told by the automated message that I'm number 12 in the queue. The emergency bypass line wasn't active today; thus, I had the displeasure of listening to the endless jingle on the phoneline for the best part of another hour while I frantically typed up my notes under the time constraints.

Saturday, 26th March 2022

The cost of living has dramatically increased. Gas, fuel, and energy prices are included. The rise in petrol prices is a big negative to our financial pockets, no thanks to the Russian invasion of Ukraine. Fortunately, the travel expenses in my team have improved from 56 pence to 66 pence per mile; however, the pay received from NHS workers is falling miles behind as the general cost of living skyrockets. Thank goodness my parents still put up with me. Affording a one-bedroom property with three years' savings seems unattainable. It's another reminder of the impact of inflation following the damages to the economy that the pandemic has already caused. Instead of saving up a decent deposit for an extortionate mortgage, I'm beginning to consider that renting is the way forward to allow more freedom and independence in my life, even though mortgage advocates say that this is just like pissing your money against the wall. But even renting is getting overpriced, and in my local area, there's a lack of options available for tenancy due to the challenges of the property market.

Monday, 26th April 2022

The place I've visited most often over the last few years has been that landscape of a beach somewhere exotic. It's the screensaver of the desktop computer in our office. Very nice indeed…

Thursday, 19th May 2022

Every community nurse in our service has a smartcard, which we insert into our work laptops, enabling us to log into our computer software and complete our documentation. Frustratingly, I lost my smartcard during a drunken weekend for a close mate's stag do in London. I know this as I stupidly stored it in my phone case, and I kept it there until we raved into the nightclubs of Shoreditch. I've been doing this since lanyards were prohibited due to possible exposure to COVID, but now lanyards have been reinstated.

Even though the stag's celebratory night out was on Saturday, I was still feeling the effects on Monday morning with symptoms of laryngitis, but luckily, the hoarse voice and sore throat are gradually easing now. I wasn't honest with my colleagues about how I lost my card; I just said that I must've misplaced it at home, but I wouldn't be surprised if some people put two and two together. I contacted the smartcard services about the issue of my missing card, and they deactivated my lost card and organised for a fresh one to be re-issued. I got it collected by the local smartcard champion today. Over the last few days, I've realised how beneficial having the mobile app for my documentation is. I don't just upload my up-to-date wound photos there and update the relevant risk assessments and care plans. I've also started dictating my progress notes rather than typing them on the laptop like usual. I wish I looked closer into reading some of my notes before I validated them. The dictation changed the word "macerated" to "masturbated." Instead of saying that a patient was settled in bed on arrival, it interpreted it as "on arrival, the patient was lying dead but appeared to be well in himself." Yes, there are still faults with twenty-first-century technology. Still, no-one can deny that it's come a heck of a long way, principally in changing the efficiency of how many jobs can be performed. We nurses are now realising how vital the mobile app is for our endless documentation.

Friday, 10th June 2022

I visited a patient today who reached 100 years old two weeks ago. He received the letter from the Queen, which he proudly displayed on his windowsill. He has hearing and visual impairments that require me to write messages on a notepad in bold letters for him to read. The cause of the deafness was due to being blown up in a tank during the war, and you can clearly see that a piece of his right ear is missing, a noticeable feature when he turned his head to have his temperature checked by my tympanic thermometer.

Despite those slight limitations, apart from atrial fibrillation and chronic kidney disease in the GP's clinical summary, he doesn't have much medical background. He's still up and mobilising with a urethral catheter attached to the leg, which is being well maintained. I even took his blood pressure today, which was better than mine. This heroic gentleman's blood pressure was 120/65. When I had mine checked by another nurse in the office the other day, it was 145/80. A bit higher than usual, but I put that down to the stress of finding the perfect apartment for me, as I'm single at 30 and flying from my family nest, hoping that the savings I've built up over the years will meet the demands of the monthly mortgage or rent costs, utility bills and other increased expenses in a cost-of-living crisis.

I'm looking at this elderly gentleman, and I couldn't imagine the amount of stress his much younger self must've gone through when he fought for our country. And yet, he has a perfect score with all his physical observation readings. I had the honour of caring for the former oldest man in the world, and I think this other gentleman today is destined to achieve that same milestone.

Wednesday, 15th June 2022

Fit testing on one of the hottest days of the year so far. I might flake away towards the end of this 45-minute-long session, with my face claustrophobic in a tight compacted space and my entire body within the stuffy boxed room with the assessor commanding ridiculous instructions at me. The same commands I heard in late November last year led to me not even wearing a single FPP3 mask on a home visit. I thought, "Is it even necessary to consider wearing these now when most of our community nurses have been managing to visit our patients with level two PPE all through the pandemic?"

Besides, it appears we're getting COVID under control, albeit the neighbour across my road almost died of it last month after a three-month-long stay in two different hospitals and three possible diagnoses of mesothelioma, kidney disease and heart failure before confirming it was the invisible killer to blame to the frightened and exhausted 70-year-old gentleman. One of the community sisters in our service is currently off work and enduring their second bout of the bastard.

Nonetheless, today does give me extra empathy for and appreciation of those on our NHS frontline who wore sufficient protection in the most challenging conditions and times of our history and for an exhausting period that still lingers. Based on the stories I've learned in the high acuity settings, my admiration for these fighting angels of our NHS was already huge. But this morning was just another gentle reminder of how brave and important they've been in treating our most vulnerable.

CHAPTER 10
AWAY FROM THE SHADOWS

Monday, 14th February 2022

When I first visit a patient of concern who's recently been referred to our service, countless thoughts spring into mind. The most common ones are whether the helpless individual is hungry, in pain or frightened. Today was no different when I spoke through the letterbox to a service user with severe depression and compulsive obsessive disorder who never leaves his flat and doesn't like visitors. He took the key out of his lockbox this week, so I couldn't let myself in. After plenty of reassurance, 58-year-old Harold allowed me in if I'd be quick. I'm glad it didn't get to the point of being on my knees, almost pleading to check the patient's bottom. It's a similar situation to other non-compliant individuals who the nurses need to review when they have a deteriorating pressure sore. How unfathomable this would look and sound to a bystander inside the block of flats, especially on this day and what it represents.

As soon as I entered, I got one massive shock. If there were an award for the most unkempt flat, it would be this one. Old urine bottles lying around needed to be incinerated in the hospital's crematorium. There were cat faeces on the floor, undoubtedly human faeces on the floor, blocks of chocolate, and other darkened, unidentifiable objects matted into the already grey and brown coloured carpet, with the dust, hair, and fur. The reason for noting human faeces was apparent. The toilet was clogged up, and Harold never wanted to get it fixed. He cared more about his cat, who he left a tray of litter out for, but obviously, the cat didn't 'give a shit' about where it was excreting either. Harold was always too intoxicated to realise the shambles around him due to his progressive alcohol-induced brain damage. Amongst all this mess on the lounge floor lay a copious amount of empty beer cans building up around the sides of his sofa chair. One day, I counted 10 cans of special brew; another day, I counted 12 cans of Stella Artois. The record number of cans I counted on a visit was 21 of 1664 Kronenburg. The house reeked of second-hand smoke, too. Yep, you guessed it, he's a chain smoker and a raging alcoholic. We ensured that the allocated nurse entered Harold's flat last on the list so that the uniform didn't get cross-contaminated in our office or another vulnerable patient's home and was shoved straight into the nurse's washing machine.

Unfortunately, you'd still be smelling and tasting the murky air from that flat as you drive home, which had been screened through the fabric of our face masks for the best part of an hour. We shouldn't blame Harold for this catastrophic situation. We've learnt from his records that he was an intelligent man with a promising career ahead of him in his younger years. In one visit with a nurse, he could remember (in perhaps a less drunken state) that he graduated from the University of Hull and was a journalist for the BBC at the heights of his life. We wonder whether something of personal devastation led to a severe mental setback between then and now, along with the multiple diagnoses affecting physical health, including swelled-up legs with leaky ulcers, type two diabetes, and a fatty, sluggish liver. A poor diet can lead to diabetes. On top of that, excessive drinking and smoking can lead to atherosclerosis, which is the thickening and hardening of the arteries due to plaque build-up – made up of fatty deposits, cholesterol, cellular waste products, calcium, and fibrin – a protein that causes blood clotting. Atherosclerosis can lead to poor circulation and heart problems, and if arteries get completely obstructed, this will lead to the acute event of a stroke or cardiac arrest.

On the evaluation of Harold's medical history, he's also lived through many years of self-neglect, no doubt causing him a great deal of insanity, and he's turned away from all social contacts he's ever developed through life. All except one person he had connections with at a charity church service. With good intentions, this Samaritan has offered anything of affordable purchases that Harold has ever wanted regularly each week. Much of the contents bought, though, is what's kept the unhealthy habits alive. An endless supply of beer, fags, and chocolate.

Wednesday, 16th March 2022

Eventually, with routine MDT meetings and a strong emphasis on Adult Services, it was agreed that Harold would be evicted from his house and admitted to the nearest mental health institute for Harold to undergo a strict detox regime. The GP recently did a memory assessment with Harold to check whether he still had the mental capacity to make his own decisions. This wasn't the case, and Harold failed to understand, retain, weigh up and communicate the correct answers, and he didn't recall what day, month, or year we were in. The good Samaritan from the local church is the only other person associated with Harold's life who's classed as the next of kin, but he's not the lasting power of attorney to make decisions in Harold's best interests. The friend still contributed to what was decided in extensive MDT meetings.

The detox regime will involve dwindling down the levels of alcohol and tobacco. Going cold turkey could lead to withdrawal symptoms, possibly even more detrimental to Harold's health. Introducing softer and clearer fluids and a balanced diet of nutrients will be the gradual replacement. This will help maintain his currently stable physical parameters.

Wednesday, 29th June 2022

Later in the year, I spotted Harold in one of our local care homes. He was sitting in one of the chairs across the lounge hall. He looked like a changed man. His hair was darker and slicker, and I could tell it was recently washed and combed. Finally, it is being handled with care and attention.

Harold had a smile when he laid eyes on me. I never thought that this guy would ever smile again after the ice-cold stares I uncomfortably encountered from him before. Even though he was persistently oblivious because of his battered brain, I could still tell he recognised me.

Nonetheless, Harold is a changed man. A happier man. Someone who feels a sense of belonging from others around him again and who's been able to restore some of his personality away from the shadows of his troubling past. It was tear-jerking and pleasing to see, and my colleagues had the same response to the delightful news I told them in the office and couldn't wait to visit him themselves. He's back on our caseload again to bring down the swelling in his legs with compression bandaging until we can get him into a pair of compression garments, which can be managed long-term now that he's no longer in an environment of self-neglect.

CHAPTER 11
AN END TO A NATIONAL TREASURE

Tuesday, 19th July 2022

Today, a UK record temperature of 40.3 degrees Celsius was recorded and verified by the Met Office in Coningsby. Spare a thought for all district nurses in this boiling weather, wearing plastic aprons, masks and gloves in the warm, confined spaces known as retirement flats. These plastic items stick to you in all the wrong places because you're moist! We drink fluids to stay hydrated and drip on the floor, washing legs and applying double-layer compression bandaging on nasty, swollen legs. Another time is when you're trying to manage with compression stockings, which aren't only hard to apply once the legs are greased up with cream and ointments, but you have the snowstorm of dead skin shavings to endure on removal first.

In addition, on sweltering summer days like today, I don't get much respite from the heat between visits. That's because the air conditioning system isn't functioning properly in my car, and it's something I'll request to get fixed in my upcoming MOT and servicing that I've booked. For now, though, I'll be roasting on these blistering days, especially when there's little shade within the miles of the patients' houses.

Thursday, 28th July 2022

I've just been on a retreat in the New Forest this week. I decided to book it spontaneously to take my mind away from the hustle and bustle of a busy life. There were various classes that I could pre-book before attending the retreat, and on the first evening, I did a spirituality talking session. The group discussion went through some interesting connections with spirituality in our lives, and one of these concepts was synchronicity; having moments that were meant to be. For example, meeting someone that made you feel tremendous. The group leader believed we were all meant to join each other for the evening. Synchronicity can resonate with people who are where they want to be in life with good fortune, and perhaps this idea doesn't echo for people facing dark times in life. Some people believe that their lives are mapped out and that God has a plan for each of us.

I also booked a couple of yoga sessions this week, where we were doing the lunged stretch pose while ensuring the tailbone stays central. Keep the legs straight first, then bend forward with the face, chest and arms reaching out in front and then toward the ceiling. Other yoga stretches included the cobra and the bridge stretch. I could see the experienced participants looking at me, thinking, "You're not elegant at all" and "You need more lessons." Evidently, the yoga class was too intense for me. I was sweating loads, partly due to how difficult the activities were for my limited flexibility, but also partly from my prostatitis that was undiagnosed at the time until I went to the doctors for a consultation, blood tests, and a urine sample smelled like rotting fish, which it had done for the past week with difficulty to pee. All this happened during my 'relaxation' at the retreat, along with throbbing aches and pains in my head, all four limbs and stomach. These symptoms were a lot more emphasised when lying in bed overnight.

The yoga instructor in both my sessions could see me struggle and said, "If you need to stop at any point, just stop," but I persevered like the trooper that I am, even though the bending down wasn't helping with my pounding headaches and standing up again gave me a sense of light-headedness, and I could only move with pigeon steps on the mat to stabilise myself. The yoga was very challenging, and in hindsight, I should have started on a beginner's course to avoid the embarrassment of needing the blocks and straps for help among the independent 40-to-60-year-olds. So, it's safe to say I didn't get the ideal restoration from the retreat, costing £100 per night with the additional fees of the therapy sessions and classes; unfortunately, it wasn't money well spent.

Thursday, 4th August 2022

The Bank of England increased interest rates again from 1.25% to 1.75% as it battles to curb rising prices. It's the biggest rise in 27 years and will intensify the pressure on households already struggling with the cost of living. Although it increases the return on savings accounts, it makes mortgages and loans more expensive, and ultimately, I won't be able to go property hunting any time soon. I realise I have much to be grateful for still. I have my health and my parents, who've kept a roof over my head and allowed me to continue to save up well due to low rent in the hope of keeping my dream alive of a future with more independence and achieving those life goals we set ourselves in adulthood. I stay optimistic, though, that there will be a crash in the property market, which will surely make homes affordable for the hardworking people of my generation. I think it's more likely for this country to hit a recession first. I hope I'm wrong.

Wednesday, 14th September 2022

I visited London to pay my respects following the death of Queen Elizabeth II. The nation has been mourning her loss for the past week. Her face is always on the TV, every hour of the day, about her life in the Royal family, her coronation on becoming Queen at age 25, and she's graciously represented our country with a welcoming smile. The people adored her in their thousands, including those who greeted the coffin through Buckingham Palace to Westminster Abbey today.

It's been perplexing to get my head around the recent events; it still feels surreal and longer than six days ago when the Queen passed away. It was amazing to hear that my brother, Tom, could pay his respects to the Queen beside the coffin in St Giles' Cathedral. He lives in Edinburgh, takes up the once-in-a-lifetime opportunity, and waited five hours until he was given the nod to enter. This historical event is something that none of us will forget. Even though Chris, Mum and I didn't see the Queen's coffin today, we were completely overwhelmed and amazed by the endless amounts of cards and flowers people had left for her. Not forgetting the marmalade sandwiches put into a bag with a note that read, "This is for later." It put into perspective how special the Queen was and how she touched so many lives, dedicating 70 years of her life to providing a remarkable service to her nation's people whilst on the throne.

In her final hours at her holiday home in Balmoral, I'd like to think that she found comfort in Prince Charles, her noble son, in becoming King Charles III, and she was reassured in knowing that all her forthcoming duties are to be in good hands. And that Her Royal Highness will be welcomed into heaven with her beloved Prince Philip, his Lillibet.

Tuesday, 20th September 2022

We often visit infirm service users of elderly ages, which correlates to an ever-growing and ever-ageing population. We know that for many of these patients their time is short with us, but today was still a bit of a shock to hear that one of our patients with a complex wound had suddenly died at night. Wilfred was an 87-year-old who was hemiplegic and debilitated following a stroke. He was rigged up to four litres of home oxygen, and it was on the cards that he was becoming end of life. Fortunately, the GP had made contact within the month, and the patient was treated palliatively with a catheter in situ since he became doubly incontinent with all care on the bed, and the introduction of high-calorie supplements to replace the mouthfuls of food that he was turning his nose up at. Wilfred had a gaping category four wound. You can refer to chapter three of my previous book about the meaning of this term. It's the worst degree of pressure injury, and for Wilfred's wound, there was undermining of between three-to-six centimetres on each angle measured by a wound probe.

The one positive was that the wound was mostly clean with healthy red granulation tissue, which we wanted. When the granulation is a tomato or strawberry jam colour, that's healthy-looking; however, if it's a dark raspberry colour, it's not so good and may indicate infection. But there was also a small white area at the bottom of the cavity and in the centre of the wound bed, which was bone. Therefore, Wilfred was at high risk of osteomyelitis. The TVNs had decided a couple of weeks ago to commence topical negative pressure (TNP) therapy; a dressing with tubing connected to a pump to provide a vacuum effect. Since the rising cost of living, we've noticed scepticism from people requiring electrical medical equipment, including an airflow mattress that runs 24-hourly. The cost of running these appliances in a household is a matter of pennies per day, and the pump operating these vacuum-assisted dressings uses less energy than boiling a kettle and approximately the same power as charging an iPhone, according to the manufacturers. Even though we knew we wouldn't heal Wilfred's wound while he was alive, we still had to manage symptoms of high exudate constantly oozing. The TNP therapy is effective in suctioning fluids from chronic and static wounds that have depth and remove possible infections.

We suggested that the GP prescribe prophylactic antibiotics because of the elevated risk of wound infection. That's despite the physical observations taken each visit, which weren't too alarming, apart from consistently low blood pressure, even up until my last appointment with Wilfred yesterday, the day of the Queen's funeral.

And yes, I had to work on the bank holiday, but I didn't mind. The extra money helped, and I saw glimpses of the ceremony throughout the day with every household I went to.

While I was with Wilfred during that momentous service on TV, I realised how much Wilfred adored the Queen. The daughter explained before how Wilfred worked over at Mount Batten. The Queen would regularly visit the chicken farm, often occupied by Wilfred, who managed to pick some of the finest eggs, and he'd see how the hens and the roosters were doing. A time in Wilfred's life that he treasured, I'm sure. The live-in carers decided to switch off the footage of the funeral day in Wilfred's bedroom while I was there, and Wilfred was slumped on his right side on his hospital bed, disengaged with anything happening around him. I have a sneaky suspicion that the death of a beloved person in his life was the last nudge he needed to pass over to the other side with Her Majesty.

CHAPTER 12
THE DEMAND FOR BETTER PAY

Monday, 10th October 2022

We celebrate and recognise World Mental Health Day on this day every year. It made me think to myself: we always ask our service users how they feel, and with their consent, we can suggest mental health referrals to them, which we will do via the GP if we consider that this can benefit the patient's psychological well-being. But I believe that staff never really talk about how they feel within their teams, even in their personal life with friends and family who they trust.

Research shows that over £2 billion is the annual cost to the NHS for toxic behaviour in the workplace, causing staff to have sick leave, tap into mental health support services, and even leave for good. It's alarming when we see the figures of staff leaving the NHS due to stress and feeling at breaking point. The suicide rates of healthcare professionals can be more worrying. The global pandemic that we've recently endured won't help matters. In a recent training that I attended on compassionate leadership, the lecturer showed us a graph. It displayed a wavy line projecting upwards, and it identified that in the post-COVID-19 pandemic, there's already a tsunami of people suffering from stress, anxiety and depression at high rates. The lecturer warned that this line on the graph would linger at an elevated level for several years because this human behaviour repeats itself after a pandemic occurs every 100 years.

Knowing this information made me realise that people are dying not only because we live in a darker world but because people are rude to each other. Simple. You cannot tell people to be nicer, but as a compassionate leader, you can lay the foundations to make people feel safe, included, valued and confident to speak up. In a team, you can ask how each other's day was. You can ask if anyone is feeling dehydrated and needing a drink. Does someone need a debrief after a traumatic incident?

We all have grey days when taking ourselves in to work is difficult. We all have our own lives away from our jobs, which sometimes gets too much. It can even be personal health problems. The menopausal symptoms for female nurses include hot flushes, night sweats and difficulty sleeping. This stage of life can be very challenging and can impact a number of things, including employment.

We must acknowledge when bad times affect our working mentality and the quality of our care and seek help when needed. Informing your matron or other line managers is the first step to this, and you may need time out to contact your support network until you feel strong enough to work again. You shouldn't feel like you're a nuisance for speaking out about this because if nothing is done to help yourself out, then your issues can manifest until you reach a crisis, resulting in a longer time out to heal your poor health and well-being status and your nursing service will have a prolonged absence of the wonderful, compassionate care that you provide.

Monday, 17th October 2022

Can you 'pop in?' This question is one of our pet hates as a community nurse when it comes from the GP or another service. It sounds like we're on a TV programme and need to get the push bike out. A scary four-word question that you don't want to hear from the triage nurse or the hospital ward discharging a patient because you know that sometimes this won't be a quick in-and-out job. Today was no different.

Firstly, I see in the triage notes that he lives at "The Farm." The weather has been atrocious, and I only washed and cleaned my car at the weekend. That was a waste of time now. I also couldn't fathom where the address was first for love nor money, and the sat-nav in my car didn't register the postcode of this remote area.

The notes said the wound on the patient's leg was "just a little scratch" where he knocked it. I then arrive and follow the trail of blood from the lobby to the kitchen and then the lounge, where the patient is slumped to one side on the settee. I was surprised that he had a gash on his forehead and a patch of skin on their right lower leg hanging off. Bonus points for dried kitchen roll stuck to the wound, too! He clearly took a nasty tumble, and these deep gashes needed more than just a first-aid patch-up job. I needed to call for the paramedics to get their stitching kit out and potentially send the poor man into the hospital with a blood transfusion after the total volume he'd lost. I tied a dark-coloured hand towel around the bloody area of the damaged leg to act as compression, and I also applied an iodine dressing and an absorbent pad to the trauma site on the head before wrapping a few layers of soft bandaging around the head to stop the bleed. I also got him to elevate his legs, which was a good idea for him anyway, based on how swollen his ankles were. Hemosiderin staining was seen in the ankles and shin area; a brown pigmentation of iron from red blood cells where the veins get distended. It's not harmful but a permanent staining and a feature of chronic venous insufficiency. When assessing a service user, you play detective, not just by reviewing the history of medical conditions but also by checking the active medications they're on and if they have any allergies. There's a lot to consider. A penicillin allergy has cropped up many times among patients, and this fact is crucial to know about, especially if antibiotics need to be introduced at any stage. When I saw this gentleman's Dossette box today, one of his medications was Amlodipine; a calcium channel blocker used to treat hypertension. Swelling is the most common side effect of Amlodipine, usually manifesting in the feet. When looking at a clinical trial study of this drug given to thousands of patients, the amount of people experiencing swelling appears to be related to the dose taken. Hopefully, he can have a medication review with this in mind following today's hospital admission, but assessing the severity of his injuries will hold greater importance initially. The good thing with medications is that they come in variations, so there are often alternative options. I'll refer to the diuretic treatment in this gentleman's case. If a patient has swollen legs resembling one of those roly-poly, round-bottomed dolls that wobble when they move, furosemide is the first choice for effectively treating this. But if that patient's kidney function is poor, then they could try bumetanide, which is also a diuretic and can work as an antihypertensive and is metabolised by the liver instead.

Wednesday, 2nd November 2022

I posted my vote for industrial strike action a couple of weeks ago, and the deadline was today. The fact that the RCN (the chief nursing trade union) have put in a big dispute for the pay of the professionals it represents will mean that there will no doubt be a backlash. My colleagues and I are becoming aware that in the next few weeks, a lot of bad press will be fired at nurses and many others who work within the NHS. For those who don't work in healthcare, there are some alarming facts that nursing staff have had to deal with and struggle through, specifically in the most recent years.

Fortunately, when I took on my post-graduate degree in nursing, there was no tuition fee to pay, but I've remained in debt from my undergraduate sports degree, which started at just over £20k. In 2022/23, a newly qualified nurse who leaves university will have an average student debt of £35,000. This means that nine per cent of their gross salary will be taken monthly in student loan repayments. A nine per cent deduction will likely continue for the majority of these newly qualified professionals' lives until it's written off after 30 years. For a registered nurse in the NHS, the starting salary now is £27,055. When you begin nursing, a series of financial deductions will sting you. You'll pay the compulsory £120 for registration to the Nursing and Midwifery Council (NMC) to practice every year. An unlucky number of nurses will pay between £200-500 per year in parking fees (depending on the Trust they work for) before even stepping through their hospital or workplace door. They'll pay £15-£20 per month for union membership and professional indemnity. Breaks for a nurse are unpaid. A nurse is entitled to two 30-minute breaks per long day (for a 13-hour shift) if you can find the time in your busy schedule to catch your breath!

The Demand for Better Pay

The Guardian has published an analysis from Thinktank and GMB, which establishes the shocking scale of pay cuts for all professionals across the NHS after the adjustment for inflation. It shows that the real wages for a nurse and health visitor have dropped by £1583 on average per year since 2011, an average doctor's compensation has fallen by £779, and for midwives, it's dropped by £1,813. But analysing nursing separately and its pay scheme up to now across the bands, there's an average of 11% less than how the pay was worth a decade ago.

The years of underinvestment and low recruitment have raised the thousands of vacancies across the country for nursing jobs. In turn, this costs NHS services approximately £6 billion per year in expensive agency staff. This underappreciation for the profession has caused countless staff members to walk out, leaving their strained teams providing unsafe care for the growing caseload of patients. To back this up, a study found that the risk of harm increases by seven per cent for every extra patient a nurse is asked to look after beyond a safe amount.

Nurses aren't greedy. They've worked through a gruelling pandemic to help keep everyone safe. Many have sacrificed their lives for the job, with an estimated 850 deaths of healthcare workers during the pandemic. Not only that, but nurses have lost colleagues and family members to COVID-19.

My colleagues and I need not listen to the government propaganda. The latest pay deal amounted to a pay cut in real terms, and a letter from the RCN, there are other important reasons why it's time to take strike action.

Our patients aren't safe, and their safety and wellbeing are our primary concern. Still, chronic neglect of the NHS, which is on its knees, has left patients waiting dangerously long for treatment, missing care altogether and in some cases, paying the highest price because we aren't adequately staffed.

Our work isn't recognised; our roles within the nursing profession are increasingly complex, requiring levels of responsibility and specialist knowledge that should be met with far higher pay. We've been undervalued and underpaid by consecutive governments, especially when the cost of living has significantly increased, with inflation rising by 10.1% from recent data on BBC News. This vote will be pivotal in securing the respect, appreciation and renumeration that nursing deserves.

Our pay has been held down for too long. We're providing safety-critical care to the population and are the largest workforce in the NHS, and yet too many of our members are forced to use food banks and to choose between heating their homes and feeding their children hot meals. It's a national disgrace, and we shouldn't stand for it. Industrial action is a powerful tool for change.

CHAPTER 13
THE IMPORTANCE OF PATIENT CENTRED CARE

I've known Tamara since starting as a staff nurse, and her mobility was at a noticeable deficit on my first visit in early 2019. Predominantly wheelchair-bound, Tamara could still get to the kitchen swiftly on wheels with her upper body strength. Overall, it was a pleasure to work with this lady, who was a youngster at heart, playing video games in her room and keeping track of the latest blockbuster films on a blue-ray disk. Once Tamara heard my call as I entered the side door, she rolled herself from her bedroom to the kitchen, where the wound care took place. Her eyes glistened as she greeted me in her chair. During the hour I was there, we had a nice, long natter about her previous life experiences and my personal life in each visit. By the same token, my abilities in providing bilateral leg ulcer care were advancing. It was like an enjoyable workshop to add to my weekly schedule.

Tamara's neurological disease, which materialised in her 40s, has undeniably taken hold of her vocal cords. Whilst doing dressing changes, it became challenging to understand what Tamara was pronouncing during sentences. I didn't want to ask her to repeat herself too many times in case she got annoyed. I occasionally nodded with a "yes" and a smile, hoping that what she was saying at times just needed some acknowledgement and agreement.

She was suffering with pain down her legs, no thanks to the arterial damage. Tamara was prescribed amitriptyline (medication commonly used as an antidepressant) but low doses of 10 milligrams work well for neuropathic pains affecting anywhere on the body. Painful diabetic neuropathy was included in Tamara's case, and it can also work well for arterial leg ulcer patients with leg pains. As with most medications, though, it comes with side effects, and in Tamara's situation, the amitriptyline can cause drowsiness alongside the regular morphine doses.

There were multiple ulcers on both of Tamara's legs, too. They were very slow to heal, not helped by the fact that she smokes excessively daily; however, smoking cessation advice didn't seem appropriate because of Tamara's low quality of life. We can't rob her of the minimal enjoyment she still gets from life. The legs were also leaking uncontrollably with burning serous fluid, which was the reason for us visiting three times a week for many months. TVNs and vascular nurses examined Tamara's legs and investigated complications in her poorly functioned arteries, so her legs were treated palliatively. No compression therapy is suitable and will likely cut off the rest of the circulation that Tamara has in the downstairs department. Therefore, managing with conservative dressings and soft bandaging was the central option going forward.

Over a couple of years into my post, we managed to get on top of the wound care to Tamara's legs, drying up and only requiring weekly visits. The pain became more under control through the involvement of the palliative care doctor from Phyllis Tuckwell. But usually, in our job, we face the conundrum: when one problem is resolved, another problem emerges. This is the case with Tamara, as her risk of pressure sores has increased over the last two years due to her depleting mobility.

Unsurprisingly, pressure ulcers emerged on her buttocks. Her habit of sitting in the wheelchair for extended periods (because she was fixated on playing video games) was a contributory factor. This led to additional pain in the coccyx, sacrum, and natal cleft, as well as her buttocks. All these bones have importance in giving us a stable structure in a sitting position. All this pain made Tamara want to remain stationary. Sitting or lying completely still, without repositioning herself, because each twinge of movement would cause pain every time. Her partner, David, who she first met through her engineering career, has also declined in health with his rheumatoid arthritis. A gentleman who was Tamara's sidekick through her glory years and was of helpful assistance at the start of Tamara's care journey. They treasured each other's company and were now concerningly distant in a household filled with tension. David cannot now assist Tamara with standing transfers, from chair to bed, using the standing aid previously assessed as necessary by occupational therapy.

Tamara's behaviour has been challenging at times throughout our care with her. All her pent-up frustrations of an illness crippled her with her independence and quality family life. It was bound to break through the surface now and again. But Tamara's mood was consistently low when the wounds developed on her buttocks; skipping dressing changes, skipping meals, wasting away. Simply giving up. Perhaps it was also a way of showing control.

David was in turmoil and couldn't cope living with Tamara in this state. David had also lost all trust in the local GPs, who only offered e-consult and video links instead of face-to-face consultations at the house. Communication was particularly problematic at the peak of the coronavirus pandemic. Our nursing service strongly advocated David's case, and with support also through Adult services, an urgent admission to the local community hospital for respite care was decided. Tamara was strongly encouraged to go through with this as a last roll of the dice, laying on the simply brutal facts that malnourishment or sepsis would kill her sooner or later if nothing changed at home.

Monday, 31st October 2022

When I visited Tamara after her hospital stay, there was life back. Her eyes had a twinkle again. There was colour again. Her cheeks were rosy on either side. She looked fuller, with extra pounds being added to the scales. With intense involvement from the physiotherapy team on the ward, Tamara was able to bear weight on her legs with the standing transfer device for a few minutes at a time. Something that she couldn't even attempt for a good month prior to hospital due to her increased frailty. It was safe to say that, at this point, we got our Tamara back. Still, maintaining Tamara at her best will be a new challenge for the following weeks.

Friday, 4th November 2022

In the first week of returning home, Tamara refused to have an alternating airflow mattress on a hospital bed. Her reasons for this were that she claimed she was uncomfortable when resting on an airflow mattress in the hospital, and the air panels restricted her movements. The nurses who've been closely connected with Tamara had suspected there was a more meaningful motive. In a tearful visit with Tamara, she emotionally spoke out that lying on a hospital bed would remind her of when she was at her lowest and believed that she was sent home to die on such equipment.

Friday, 11th November 2022

Through a short space of time, we've managed to rewire Tamara's mindset that having a pressure-relieving mattress on a profiling bed will be an excellent thing, alongside adequate nutritional intake. When the ulcerated legs had leaked profusely before, Tamara's albumin levels were noticeably reducing. Albumin is a protein the liver makes and can be monitored with routine blood tests. Normal albumin levels are 35-to-50 grams per litre, but if the numbers get too low, which they did for Tamara because she was losing more protein in the wound exudate, the body won't have enough sources of protein to aid wound healing.

Thankfully, the leg ulcers healed at this stage. Much of this was down to constant leg elevation during the hospital (which we know from a previous story has significant benefits at sending blood from the peripheries of the legs back to the heart). We face less risk of Tamara's albumin decreasing, and our nutritional advice included the encouragement of fortified drinks prescribed by the pharmacy, which are rich in protein. Tamara was on board with these alongside her usual diet.

We reminded Tamara that her condition had improved immensely in just three weeks. Her humour and personality were getting restored at that time when she thought she was going to die at the start. Following her acceptance of appropriate equipment and the addition of a carer visiting four times a day to support her with chair-to-bed transfers and toileting needs, the bottom sores were fading away like the leg ulcers. With Christmas approaching, Tamara no longer has bandaging on her legs from the base of her toes to just below knee level, which she relied on for several years. Instead, Tamara can wear her pairs of fluffy stripey socks. We've reached our desired outcome with Tamara because our holistic approach with her enabled successful patient-centred care. It provided the intrinsic benefit of respecting the individual's feelings and values, and it led to improved behaviours and compliance.

CHAPTER 14
THE UNEXPECTED APPOINTMENT

Monday, 14th November 2022

Today, I started my new position as an Enhanced Wound Care Nurse. It's a role implemented across community nursing teams in recent years because there's a growing need to effectively facilitate the care of our patients who require wound care. I'll be looking to case-manage and aid an efficient delivery of care, delegating with my new team members and guided by carefully organised wound care regimes. Leg ulcers between the knee and ankle joint, unhealed for at least two to four weeks, are the most common wounds we see. Approximately 1.5% of the UK's adult population is affected by active leg and foot ulceration, equating to 730,000. Only 16% of lower leg wounds have a diagnosis, which tells me that nursing services need to do more Doppler assessments to get patients into the most suitable form of treatment and to heal legs at the quickest rates; a key area I'll look to prioritise.

Monday, 28th November 2022

Referring to the lone worker policy, if we feel like we're at risk of harm in a patient's home, it's been advised to contact a senior or colleague on our phone to tell them we're going to be late home and to ask them to "feed my dog." By saying those three words, that phrase should signify to the receiver that we're in potential danger. The receiver should then ask questions that require "yes" or "no" answers to discover more about the situation and alert the police. This is when our emotional intelligence comes into play, as it should come across as a casual conversation over the phone so the service user doesn't suspect anything.

That phrase to help with de-escalation is becoming obsolete as staff have now been given lone-worker devices. They're small, black, chargeable devices attached to our lanyards, and we're instructed to press the SOS button to alert the security department. Once they get responses to their "yes" or "no" questions, they can filter that information instantly to the police, and the GPS tracker programmed into the mini machines can pinpoint exactly where we are.

The Clinical Services manager has also informed us to deactivate our devices when out of hours. There was a false activation of a device at the weekend and a subsequent telephone call with a security manager to an embarrassed and somewhat tipsy clinician who kept the device in their pocket on a night out after their shift had finished. I imagine they didn't wear their full uniform to the pub, but the company monitoring these alarms and who organised the escalation processes wasn't best pleased, and an awkward chat between the culprit and the shift lead undoubtedly occurred this morning.

Wednesday, 30th November 2022

I went with a TVN to a redundant hotel for a clinical appointment. The TVN proposed the visit to me this morning as a unique learning experience that'll involve a translator to help. The temporary service user was referred to us by a paramedic, who was a warden of the hotel alongside a group of other lovely, attentive paramedics. This young patient was a refugee living in the hotel with other men of young adult ages. The paramedic warned us that these refugees may feel agitated and resentful for being confined in separate rooms in this joyless, darkened building. Therefore, I supported the TVN with someone who was potentially hostile yet didn't speak a word of English. The refugee was referred under the watchful eye of the wound care specialists because he sustained multiple leg ulcers. These citizens of Afghanistan were forced to flee their country because of wars, persecution, torture or genocide. Many have been and continue to be housed in bridging hotels like the one I visited this afternoon.

Before entering the facility, the paramedic discussed how the leg ulcers were sustained. The refugee escaped from the awful conditions of his homeland in Afghanistan. He did it by boat, and unfortunately on his way over to the UK, his boat capsized but he miraculously survived and got onto UK shores. When he was found, he was admitted to a hospital and sent to A&E. It was suspected from the medical assessments that he'd been emersed in water for several hours and in the process of being pushed along by the ocean currents, his legs smashed into rocks and boulders until he was pulled through and hit land. The same TVN first saw the refugee a couple of weeks ago, and his legs were in a nasty state, with some of the gashes measuring a centimetre deep, and they were traumatic with bleeds.

According to recent data from the UK Home Office, Afghans are the largest nationality of small-boat immigrants, followed by Indians. It must be a perilous journey for people like him, who fled their hometown after a final goodbye to family in an attempt to reach the English shore by sea, especially since the police have cracked down on those crossing illegally by train, lorry or car. The reason for doing this is to claim asylum; an application for international protection for fear of being returned to their own country or origin of residence.

After plonking our medical appliances onto a chair and creating a sterile field with our dressing packs on a table in a lounge area of the hotel, in stepped the refugee accompanied by a paramedic. He resembled a teenager with dark, shaggy hair, no facial hair and wearing an orange t-shirt and black sports shorts. This young lad sheepishly walked further into the room wearing sandals on a cold December day outside. He then sat on a chair while the TVN grabbed another chair and sat opposite him. The other medic with us then contacted the translator on mobile, who could speak English and Dari Persian, which the refugee speaks and is the most common language spoken in Afghanistan.

During an appointment as unique as this, with the addition of a member of the telephone translation services, the linguist (human and non-robotic) waits until the speaker (either me, the TVN or the refugee) has finished converting what was said from one language to another. The refugee's legs had several beige-coloured dressings on all angles. After some small talk going back and forth, the TVN addressed that she'd like him to wear compression stockings on his legs after today's visit to help heal the legs quicker, but to do that, he'll need to have his circulation checked with the use of a clever machine. The refugee was on board with this and agreed to lie on the floor in the middle of the room. I was surprised how agreeable he was to do this, without us having to rationalise that lying flat for 20 minutes settles the systemic blood pressure and improves the accuracy of the vascular assessment.

Usually for these tests, I use a handheld Doppler probe (as previously explained), but today I used a machine that's evolved from that device, called a MESI. Whenever I hear this name, I think about one of the greatest footballers on the planet, Lionel Messi. The pleasing thing with the MESI machine is that it speedily records the measurements of a patient's suitability for compression once the wired-up blood pressure cuffs on both ankles and the arm with (the highest systolic pressure) inflate and deflate in a synchronised manner and a matter of a couple of minutes.

"Your arm and legs will tighten up for a few seconds, but try not to move and you'll be OK," I said. Once the message was translated over the phone, the refugee lifted his head slightly, and he gave me a thumbs up with a half-smile.

While kneeling over him and hooking him up to the medical appliance, I couldn't take his angelic looks at face value; for he may be a person with ideologies that pose a threat of terrorism. He may have similar feelings to those who've plotted an attack on our country, just like the four suicide bombers who performed al-Qaeda-inspired attacks and killed 52 people across the London transport system on the 7th of July 2005. That's why the local authorities don't treat these refugees well, and aren't allowed to stay in one place for too long to get comfortable and make friends. That's why they're being moved around from place to location, to stay in remote areas and in unwanted buildings to try and make them feel uneasy in the hope of shutting down the chances of more refugees coming over.

I still felt some degree of sympathy for this young person. He must've encountered such horrible events in his own country to make him travel in such risky circumstances. Does he have a mum or a dad or any siblings? Does he know of someone that loves and cares about him? No name and date of birth ending in 1997, which didn't seem right, but the paramedic addressed in the introductory stage of the visit that dates of birth can be forged to make people appear older to have more of a privilege of independent living. It must've been horrific enough for him to try and survive in deep water in desperation. I wonder if he or others in his situation will suffer from post-traumatic stress syndrome (PTSD) from their experiences. It's not for me to investigate. In these cases, all we can do is lift rocks and look at what might be underneath.

Once it was all finished with perfect readings on the screen of the appliance, indicating suitability for strong compression therapy, I said to the refugee with a thumb up, "All finished." The refugee lifted his head marginally, gave me a thumbs up with an open smile, and said, "Thank you." I then instructed him to sit back in the chair to receive wound care, which he was happy to proceed with. After peeling off the dressings, the wounds were drying up nicely and looked more like superficial grazes now, but I suppose he has age on his side with a quicker inflammatory response for the skin tissue to heal in comparison to the older individuals I'm normally treating. His face was a picture when the TVN dangled a pair of black compression stockings in the air and told him to wear them over the top of the new dressings. At first, he grinned and glanced down in reluctance; however, I think we won him over by the hosiery being open-toed so he could still wear his sandals, and he applied them on without any problems before waving us bye and walking back to his room with the paramedic following him. This had to be one of the most interesting and strangest clinical appointments I had been involved in.

CHAPTER 15
THE CRUELTY OF A LIFE-LIMITING CONDITION

Whilst dealing with wounds has become integral to my nursing career, I've seen how injuries can impact working lives. With younger people, it can noticeably affect their careers and relationships. It can be a vicious circle since comorbidities like stress predispose patients to non-healing wounds, often leading to disability, with psychological stressors directly impacting healing outcomes. These correlations can be highlighted in the episodes of care that we've had with Edgar, a 44-year-old and diagnosed with multiple sclerosis (MS), one of the most challenging and debilitating conditions. He was diagnosed with a primary progressive version of MS in 2006, which had rapidly accelerated since the birth of his son nine years ago. I first visited Edgar three years ago, in April 2019, due to a sacral sore he sustained from sitting in his wheelchair. Edgar was operating well in his manual wheelchair with his six-year-old boy sitting cross-legged next to him in the room, glued to children's TV programmes, before running around the lounge and the kitchen when his jolly, hyperactive mood kicked in. At my initial assessment, Edgar had routine reviews from the physiotherapy team due to two recent falls.

A couple of months later, Edgar's condition was affecting the control of his bladder, and he was suffering from frequent and recurrent urinary tract infections (UTIs). Edgar was known to the urology team, and he was awaiting Botox of the bladder and was managing his urine output with a urethral catheter. At this point, the skin on his sacrum was also becoming extremely vulnerable, and due to regular accidents from his bowels before getting to the commode in time and the occasional spillages of urine, he was not only getting pressure damage but also moisture damage to the bony prominence. My nursing team visited him at allotted times in the afternoon, fitting in with when Edgar and his wife picked up their son from school, still trying to keep up with fatherhood.

Over the next episodes of care, we noticed additional complications in Edgar's daily living, including difficulties managing his urethral catheter with his bladder spasms and signs of dysphagia. During a holistic assessment of these ongoing issues, I urgently referred the MS specialist nurse to reassess Edgar's condition. More changes happened in the four weeks that proceeded. Edgar came out of the Royal Marsden

Hospital with a suprapubic catheter to avoid further spasms and discomfort, with 40 milligrams of baclofen taken daily to help. That appeared to be working, and by the end of July 2019, the sacral wound was fully healed, and Edgar's independent repositioning in the bed and transfers from bed to wheelchair. Transfers required the support of a banana board and assistance from either his carer, who visited every morning, or his wife at other parts of the day, and this was essential because of the paralysis progressing in his lower limbs.

Monday, 1st August 2022

Almost three years later, Edgar returned to our caseload. He'd recently returned from a holiday in Cornwall with his wife and son. An eight-hour stay in his wheelchair each way of the journey deteriorated the skin integrity of his sacrum, resulting in almost category four damage, and contributed to new sores developing on his spine and left buttock. Also, Edgar was getting noticeable weight loss, not helped by his swallowing difficulty and choking risks, which started with eating finely chopped food, turning to purred food, and then fortified build-up drinks. The recent dietary changes are still causing problems with swallowing, which is regularly monitored by speech and language therapy (SALT).

Edgar now relies on physical transfers using a ceiling hoist, and he's lying on a hospital bed most of the time with an alternated air-flow mattress and a habitual positioning change from carers and his wife daily for every possible chance of effective pressure relief. Edgar is heading towards becoming bedfast and no longer being a dependable father to his son, although he knows he can still communicate moral values when necessary.

Monday, 22nd August 2022

Edgar's deterioration in swallowing consequently led to a percutaneous endoscopic gastrostomy (PEG) feeding tube being inserted through the skin and into the stomach after further analysis from SALT and a dietician to assist with feeding. The PEG feeding requires fortified liquid and, at times, water and medications to be administered through a gastronomy tube, which passes through the abdominal wall and into the patient's stomach because oral intake is no longer adequate.

Wound care has become increasingly challenging. Conservative dressing changes to debride away the necrotic and sloughy tissue, then change to spells of TNP therapy to vacuum out the unwanted fluid and bring the wound base back to its original skin level again.

Friday, 9th September 2022

Several reviews later from TVNs and Enhanced Wound Care Nurses, we still have two significant pressure ulcers present, which don't change in appearance with the left buttock wound of over four centimetres deep and with failed attempts of TNP therapy. This treatment failed because the wound was too moist for the vacuum dressing to be sealed and function effectively, and because it's in a precarious location and Edgar has regular position changes in bed for pressure relief, it was coming off far too frequently, never lasting 24 hours.

Tuesday, 20th September 2022

Edgar had already suffered urosepsis six months ago, and it's been crucial to avoid clinical signs of wound infection for this dreadfully vulnerable gentleman by following the aseptic non-touch technique. Thankfully, these wounds have gradually shown improvement, leaking less and remaining clean-looking, and Edgar has been able to leave his bed for brief periods in the daytime. He even had assisted transfers into a garden chair when the weather was warmer and brighter; however, this hasn't gone exactly to plan. After a short while of sitting in the garden, he was getting covered by tiny flies, and he couldn't even scratch his nose that they were irritating, let alone swing an arm to swish them away. So, Edgar only has hoisted transfers off his bed to sit on the supportive chair opposite the TV in the same living room.

Edgar's blood pressure lowered, making him feel a little giddy when he sat upright. Therefore, extra shots of water were now pushed through the PEG feed, and the glycerol suppository was periodically inserted to help when hardened stools were forming. The volume of the pro-source supplement was also increasing per feeding hour to compensate for the weight lost during Edgar's critical illness.

With every moving and handling operation, the wife is summoned to be present, whether a two-hourly turn in the bed is due or if Edgar calls out at the Alexa alarm system. His weakening voice still has enough strength to alert the device and make Fiona aware that Edgar would like something done when this is between the three-times-a-day visits of the carers. There's a lot for Fiona to juggle, but she still manages to work as an on-call IT technician for a local business and play a strong, playful, and supportive mother to her ever-growing son. At the same time, Edgar remains helplessly in the bed.

Fiona tells the nurses now and again that she finds everything too much and is often shutting herself away from reality by going upstairs to her study room. Fiona has difficulty sitting with Edgar in the evenings when things become much more sensitive to her. She's previously said, "I keep searching for answers, but I know deep down that there are no answers apart from the end of the disease process." Fiona's sometimes gone into depth, telling us how she's trying to cope. She occasionally speaks about her thoughts and anxieties about being a mum and a wife and struggling to see a bright future. At times, she feels trapped but cannot see how to improve the situation, just feeling like she's living one long nightmare and watching the MS gradually kill her Edgar when the disease cannot be eradicated. This big overlap of responsibilities makes her tired and weary. She can also see the circumstances negatively impacting her health. At times, Fiona feels jittery and needs to lie down in bed to relax. She had noticed some weight loss when she weighed herself this morning. In summary, despite mental health concerns of her own, Fiona doesn't want Edgar to go into a care home and worries about the financial implications of this. But with Edgar at the house, keeping a solid relationship flowing with the three of them is a struggle, especially when their son has school holidays.

Friday, 7th October 2022

Edgar has a brilliant sense of humour, and on his good days, he's chatty and always having a giggle with us. His personality is infectious, and it's clear how he was able to find married life and start raising a family at a younger, healthier age. At one stage recently, Edgar and his carer were trying to convince Fiona to assist in dying his hair purple with a Mohican haircut to reminisce the days when he was a guitarist of a punk band, which was when Fiona was an adoring fan in the crowd. This brought a smile to their faces, but Edgar thought better of it not to go through with the whacky hairstyle because "there's not enough strands of hair to work with anymore."

The wounds have been improving and showing healthy, red granulation tissue and requiring twice-weekly dressing changes to manage the moderate exudate levels; however, the general care needs have become more challenging. On occasions, the urine in the catheter bag turns darker and thicker with a risk of UTIs, and increased titrations of water are put through the PEG to try and help this. The catheter has been changed frequently because of the uncontrollable bladder spasms that lead to bypassing and sometimes expelled catheters. Muscles in the limbs have also become stiffer; therefore, the MS specialist has repeatedly reviewed baclofen usage. Unfortunately, Edgar is becoming too weak to sit out in his chair for the whole afternoon, much to the son's unhappiness, who has even less engagement with his father at a tender age where an abundance of playfulness together would happen under more normal circumstances.

Wednesday, 19th October 2022

Advancements with the multi-disciplinary team in Edgar's care, including the MS specialist, have worked together and have managed to find alternative care at a nursing home placement. Edgar has understood that this will allow his wife and son to live more of a normal life elsewhere, though not too far away from regular visits now that the COVID regulations are easing again. Edgar said that he doesn't want Fiona to keep thinking that she's a horrible person for contacting a social worker and making a move to a suitable placement possible. He knows that Fiona's heart is in the right place and always has been.

Fiona couldn't endure what was happening much longer, and something had to give. One of the final straws was seeing her husband almost choking on his own vomit, and since that incident, she was terrified that he would aspirate again. Fiona believes that this local nursing home will supply the safe care that's required for Edgar now. Edgar has become aware that he has a medical need for additional care, support, and monitoring. Fiona also trusts that the new location will enable them to reconnect into a happy family again (and we all agree).

Friday, 11th November 2022

Our nurse, Tamsin, who's visited Edgar the most in our team and developed the closest relationship with him, still arranged catchups at the nursing home. In the last meeting, Tamsin couldn't help but have a good cry with Edgar, who could barely move his hands and fingers now and battles to clear any mucous from his throat and fears that this will eventually stop him from breathing. He wished euthanasia was legalised in this country, as he'd take it.

Our matron added some input for this family by signposting them to the local hospice, which can offer some extra valuable advice on how the family can support each other and how they can still find ways to make delightful memories together and help them all cope with the transition of Edgar moving from family home to nursing home.

Edgar is initially content with the new facilities. He has been pleased with how his wounds have improved, presenting as small superficial lesions with epithelialised tissue, requiring simple band-aids and ongoing pressure relief management. Edgar hopes to access the courtyard, garden, and cinema room with his family, which will also detach him from the 'oldies.'

Tuesday, 13th December 2022

Devastating news reached the nursing office, which was filtered to me on WhatsApp since I moved offices with my new specialist wound care role. It started with a phone call from a distraught Fiona, who reported to the administration department that Edgar sadly died in hospital after being diagnosed with COVID-19. We couldn't believe how unfortunate this was for Edgar when the nursing team and care agency did so well to prevent him from being admitted to the hospital with an infection in his own home. Fiona said that when Edgar entered the hospital, his breathing became awfully weak, and he needed the life-support machine to assist. Seeing him so frail and unable to move his limbs or head at all was heartbreaking. Not only is this a reminder that COVID is still lurking, even when many deem it to be non-existent now. It's also a tragic reminder of how incredibly short life is, and this couldn't be any more truthful for those battling a life-limiting condition like Edgar.

CHAPTER 16
A WORD OF WARNING

Wednesday, 14th December 2022

It's been one month into my new development role, and I've already realised that I'll be involved in more training sessions and meetings for the extra learning required in my role and the engagement with the multidisciplinary teams. I've been noticing in Microsoft Teams meetings that there can be hideous expressions on people's faces. The picture quality can also be disruptive; people can be distorted into alien humanoids on the screen. All from the unfortunate glitches that come with technology, including people's voices being sped up after lengthy pauses, but more often, they freeze until they comprehend that no one is responding to them. This means they must sign out of the meeting room to sign back in again and proceed with their discussion. On other occasions, the speaker will sound like the Daleks from *Doctor Who*, which happens if there's bad indoor coverage or poor mobile phone reception from wherever the car is parked.

Sunday, 18th December 2022

Strikes have continued since the 15th and will continue until the 20th of December, and Ambulance services go on strike on the 21st of December. Today, I saw a startling message from an ambulance worker on a Facebook post that went viral. This long, unfiltered message started with the statement, "If this shit-show in our country carries on, we will all, as a service, as an organisation, be gone. Wholesale. It will disappear."

They said the public will end up paying for healthcare if nothing changes. Those who won't be able to afford private medical care will quite honestly get sicker and die younger. Families and children in poor neighbourhoods will be dying because they cannot receive basic medical care like antibiotics for bacterial infections while the government rakes in the profits from all the suffering.

With this message, the ambulance worker urges everyone not to buy the lies from the media about how greedy ambulance workers (and all other healthcare professionals, for that matter) are about the pay demands. They stated that it's probably the worst their service has ever been. Keeping it afloat at the cost of their well-being every single day, working typically 60–70-hour weeks. But despite the hard-working weeks, it was also claimed that the wages won't see workers through to the end of the month, yet even if the wages are sufficient, the working conditions aren't worth what they're earning.

A Word of Warning

On a busy shift for emergency workers, several call-outs can be ordered for a victim of a car crash, a house fire or a stabbing. Perhaps an unwell child or someone in need following a suicide attempt or a drug overdose. How about a confirmed cardiac arrest with CPR in progress, with the current run time being 24 minutes?

In this same alarming message, the ambulance worker adds that regardless of the skills and knowledge emergency workers have to prevent death and save lives, this is becoming an impossible task at times because all the ambulances are stuck outside the hospital stations, waiting to deliver acutely ill patients, with no indication of when the emergency vehicles will be available again.

Situations like this have been happening every day for this ambulance worker, and now they're advising everyone to get angry with the government and the mess they've left for its people financially and health-wise. There is a complete lack of respect for the NHS and the ordinary working people who deserve better, safer living.

Sunday, 1st January 2023

I've made New Year's resolutions that most other community nurses will probably break within the first month or even the first week. They're as follows:

I'll try not to look so cynical when patients tell me they're elevating their legs and going to bed at night.

But when I inspect their swelled-up legs and see strikethrough in the bandaging and dressings, this tells me another story.

I'll also aim to keep my car and boot tidy and do my best to say NO to overtime. The latter of the resolutions will be the most challenging because the main factor for falling into overtime is providing detailed documentation, which is vital in case a patient's care ever sparks concern for whatever reasons and is scrutinised below the surface. For example, suppose a service user dies unexpectedly while on our caseload. In that case, our thorough notetaking may avert us from getting into trouble if our involvement with that patient is analysed in the coroners' court. If advice is given and essential nursing interventions are provided but aren't documented, you may be considered liable for negligence or wrongdoings during the inquest procedure by witnesses who weren't present in the patient's care. It may just result in a nurse being struck off the register for suspected misconduct.

Tuesday, 3rd January 2023

More strikes are brewing. The government has offered £100 million to the NHS, but that's basically like putting a tiny band-aid on a huge gammy wound. These strikes aren't just for the poverty-stricken members of our workforce who have no option but to shop at food banks rather than supermarkets. It's for the majority of the workforce, especially in hospital settings at the moment, who enter work exhausted, knowing that they cannot give their patients the best quality of care. This isn't helped by the rise of 100,000 vacancies across the NHS board, nor the rise of patients on hospital beds with strep A infection, the common flu, and even COVID still lurking around.

Wednesday, 11th January 2023

So far, after two months, I've slotted into the role of an Enhanced Wound Care Nurse within my new team, like a glove to hand on a cold winter's day. I've also received double the number of daily emails and telephone calls compared to before. Many of these come from colleagues from the tissue viability department, either announcing upcoming training updates and conferences to help complete my new list of competencies or informing me about the latest tips and tricks in the chaotic world of wound care, which dominates the community nursing caseloads. With the advancement of the role comes greater responsibility. Now, having a closer connection to the tissue viability nurses, I need to constantly strive to help improve the productivity of the service, healing rates of wounds and get positive patient outcomes. From a business perspective, successful delivery of care will save the NHS money, especially when statistics with Medi UK in December 2022 indicated that the cost of unhealed wounds totals £8.3 billion as opposed to healed wounds costing £2.7 billion.

The skin is the biggest organ in the human body, and it has many key functions, including protection from germs, enabling the ability to sweat and regulate body temperature, allowing the metabolism of vitamin D and offering protection from ultraviolet damage. In wounds that involve full-thickness skin loss, it damages the structures of the dermis; the second skin layer, where the connective tissue is comprised of sweat glands, nerve endings, hair follicles and lymph capillaries, and these unfortunately get permanently damaged. Once the dermis is healed, it doesn't have the same structure as before and is left with scar tissue. The structures will also become vulnerable and at risk of breaking down again.

Beyond the dermis layer is the subcutaneous tissue; the lower, fatty layer of the skin. This layer has other beneficial functions, including insulation and maintaining body temperature, protecting major organs and retaining moisture in the body. Therefore, wound healing and preventing skin deterioration isn't only crucial for avoiding infection, but it also helps keep all the necessary functions that the skin provides for the human body, which will maintain homeostasis and whatever quality of life that each infirm patient is hanging onto.

Burns and surgical incisions from the hospital are usually known as acute wounds and heal in four to six weeks with primary intention; however, chronic or non-healing wounds are far more common in the community. As I'm the new point of access for my team when it comes to advice on complex wounds, I'm receiving referrals from my colleagues on a regular basis. There are three main types of chronic wounds, which I've demonstrated through stories in my earlier diary entries. These are leg ulcers (typically venous-related), pressure ulcers (the core reason being immobility) and diabetic foot ulcers (the leading cause being neuropathy).

If you type into Google how many people live in the UK with a chronic wound, it'll tell you that, based on the latest research, the figure is over 2.8 million people. In my team's caseload of patients, chronic wounds can be unknown by cause, but numerous factors contribute to why wounds become slow to heal, and this resonates again with the history of patients I've already written about. Age, diabetes, obesity, cardiovascular disease, peripheral vascular disease, lymphedema, poor nutrition, and psychological factors such as stress and depression must be considered. Other aspects that contribute to chronic wounds involve lifestyle choices. Smoking and alcohol consumption and various medications, including steroids, non-steroidal anti-inflammatory drugs, chemotherapy and other immunosuppressants, can slow wound healing.

Nelson Mandela once said, "Education is the most powerful weapon you can use to change the world."

Knowledge is power, not only to aid development in all stages of a career but in my current position. I also share wisdom with my colleagues through email, telephone chatter or handovers about the most suitable wound care at the right time. It's also imperative for nurses to share knowledge with their patients and their caregivers through our individualised care plans once face-to-face holistic assessments have been completed. These care plans will work if the service user is concordant with nursing advice and has the caregivers or an appropriate care package at home to help deliver shared care on wounds, which is often approached at the latter stages of the healing process. For instance, instructions on the daily donning and doffing of compression garments are effective in long-term preventative management once leg ulcers have healed.

We need to do our utmost to heal chronic wounds in a timely manner because they come with a great deal of inconvenience to people's lives, causing frustration, anxiety and depression and will ultimately reduce a person's quality of life. There are many consequences that patients can experience. For example, pain or discomfort, sleep disturbance, odours, and fluid leakages through dressings and clothes. Another consequence is the loss of appetite (typically due to pain, lack of sleep and wound odour). If my team is stuck between a rock and a hard place with any lingering concerns, we will contact the

A Word of Warning

TVNs, GPs, or other specialist clinicians who may know the answers to my queries.

Despite a patient's holistic aspects, dressings remain the mainstay and most accessible option for managing hard-to-heal wounds. When coming to the prime decisions of selecting the right dressing or form of treatment to help heal a certain category of wound at the best time, a nurse must turn to the relevant pathways from your local NHS trust and the wound formulary in their geographical area, as well as manufacturing advice on dressings and medical appliances, which all offer guidance when making best-practice decisions in wound management and prevention. When wound care or any other clinical procedure is undertaken by a nurse, a fundamental protocol regarding infection control precautions that we must follow and that should become second nature when delivering wound care, as well as other medical interventions, is having good hand hygiene. It promotes washing hands, using sanitiser before and after patient contact, and utilising the aseptic non-touch technique when performing clinical procedures.

In terms of dressing choices, if the wound isn't showing any warning signs of infection, then using non-medication dressings is best because they can still physically remove and reduce the bacteria and bioburden of a wound. Suppose non-medication dressings can enable the removal of necrotic debris and devitalised tissues. In that case, they can then facilitate the body's endogenous enzymes to heal these wounds because as I've mentioned in my previous book, the body heals the wound, not the dressings. As wound care nurses, it's important to know that these dressings won't kill the bacteria on a wound. When this manifests into wound infections, we've no choice but to apply our anti-microbial dressings with the introduction of antibiotics if the patient becomes systemically unwell.

We should have it in our mindset to choose anti-microbial dressings when necessary and only for the required duration because a patient can develop resistance to anti-microbial dressings, just like antibiotics. That's why we need to be careful not to overuse anti-microbial dressings. According to Antibiotic Research UK, it's estimated that 12,000 people die in the UK each year from antibiotic resistance, equivalent to the number of deaths from breast cancer, and these figures could rise to 10 million deaths by 2050 unless we make changes.

Monday, 19th January 2023

It's Time to Pay Nursing Staff Fairly
Staff Shortages Cost Lives
Clapping is Not Enough
If You Pay Fairly, Nurses Will Stay
Support Nurses and Defend the NHS
You Gave Us No Choice

A Word of Warning

These are important messages seen and heard by nurses on the picket lines over the last couple of days in the second spell of industrial action. It was a freezing cold day, but I wrapped up warm with other nurses with a picket in hand and a coffee in the other. In the afternoon, I continue my temporary withdrawal from service but with the warmth of home. I'm a member of the RCN, and I said YES to striking. There was a feeling of guilt not seeing my patients today, and I'm sure my colleagues felt the same who decided not to attend work due to striking. But the government needs to hear the voices of nurses and the NHS. Enough is enough, and the service needs to run better. A big way of achieving that is through better pay, which should improve the retention of existing staff and entice future nurses to join this magnificent service!

CHAPTER 17
WORKING IN PARTNERSHIP WITH RESIDENTIAL HOMES

Monday, 23rd January 2023

I still see many inappropriate referrals on our already stretched caseload. Not that it should be any of my business, but they should keep a file of these as prime examples of knowing when to reject them. For instance, a new referral was allocated to a staff member today. The patient is mobile and self-caring and has demonstrated that she can empty the urine bag attached to her catheter and put a night bag on it. The task for the nurse was to observe the patient putting the night bag on…

We need to go back to being more ruthless when triaging during the height of COVID-19. It's uncanny how people in the community kept quiet during 2020 when plenty of shared care was getting done between patient and caregiver. We shouldn't shy away from initiating shared care now we've moved away from a global pandemic.

I put residents from a care home on shared care today, albeit they just had a small skin tear each; one on an arm and another on a leg. Still, by getting the carers to send in a photo of their wounds and we advise what they need to do from the office over the next two to three weeks until healed, it'll save thirty minutes of a nurse's time to visit in person, deliver the wound care, write the progress notes, and forward plan other appointments. Time is precious for a nurse, so any time we can save ourselves can only be a good thing, right?

Thursday, 26th January 2023

Our lovely veteran nurse in the team retracted her retirement for another 10 years. We said she was crazy and that she should work at a slower pace in one of the local coffee shops. We're all grateful for her wonderful service, even if her working hours are halved. It's the kind-hearted nurses like her and those who redeployed out of retirement to help in the pandemic that'll keep our organisation afloat with a sense of togetherness.

Monday, 30th January 2023

Regarding referrals, you just know it'll be a matter of time before you receive your next out-of-the-blue referral from a residential home, and it's anyone's guess whether it'll be a simple task or something serious and complex. Now, this chapter isn't about criticising the functionality

Working in Partnership with Residential Homes

of care homes because they're a crucial part of helping our service run because all these facilities combined look after a considerable percentage of service users on our caseload and enable a decent opportunity to initiate shared care; an effective style of care I've previously elucidated. This section is more about mentioning the occasional unpredictability of working in partnership with residential homes.

Today was one of those days. While I was doing my round of visiting several patients in a single care home, I hurried over to see another resident who wasn't on my list and didn't have an active referral with us. The senior carer explained that the lady of concern used a hot water bottle, and overnight it got cold, so the resident buzzed and asked one of the night duty carers to refill the bottle. The foreign carer wasn't adept with the safety guidelines when managing a hot water bottle, and they filled the bottle with pure boiling water and didn't allow it to stand. At least they remembered to put the furry cover back on it.

Unfortunately, the damage was done on the left hip and abdominal area, revealing a large serous-filled blister with faint redness to the surrounding skin. It was caught early as the poor lady yelped in pain on her bed, much to the foreign carer's shamefulness. She's been groaning, rocking forward and back in her armchair to gain comfort. I advised the care home manager to enter an incident report to Adult safeguarding as the harm was inflicted on the resident, albeit in error. I also made one, stating that the injury was caused by a care worker outside of our NHS Trust.

When a burn wound is sustained, whether it's a scald through the spilling of hot liquids, contacting a hot object like a steaming iron, or some type of electrical, chemical, or flame burn, you must act fast. In the first aid advice for burns given by a Salisbury burns specialist at a wound care conference, you need to stop the burning process first. To give credit to the care staff at the accommodation, they removed the lady's nightie to expose the burn site. You need to then cool the burn, generally by running it under cool/neutral water, and the care staff did this by using a clean, soaked flannel. Analgesia was also given as this injury was undoubtedly painful. The resident was already taking codeine for her rheumatoid arthritis, but I advised regular paracetamol in combination to help take the edge off.

The burn wound was cool enough to provide wound care when I arrived, and based on recommendations from the wound formulary booklet, I dressed it with a moist, sterile gauze dressing, then a secondary absorbent dressing, making sure the adhesive border wasn't sticking to the sore aggravated skin. The burns specialist at the conference emphasised that a burn should be cooled down before dressing application, especially if cling film was to be used, because if it isn't cool, the dressing will conduct the heat from the wound, creating an oven effect and will inevitably make the injury worse, and increasing the chances of life-lasting stain on the body with scar tissue once the specialists have done all they can.

In an ideal world, we'd want these sorts of wounds to heal by two weeks to avoid scarring and loss of function to the affected limb or location on the body, and this should be the case for the resident today as her injury is categorised as superficial. But realistically, for burns causing deeper thickness skin loss, the healing time can be 21 days or more and for full-thickness skin loss, there are high chances of surgery being needed prior to the healing process. By surgery, I mean skin grafting, and the specialist team would be looking for the dead and devitalised skin tissue to dry out first, and generally, the skin grafting will be taken from the buttocks or thighs.

When I reflect on previous standout moments at residential homes, I go back to a couple of cases of residents being identified as having maggot-infested wounds. These weren't the organic kind of larvae either, specially bred to be sterile to prevent infection, applied into a gaping wound inside a bio bag, which is like a tea bag, and they usually stay in place for five days. Medically used larvae is used to remove necrotic, sloughy, and infected tissue. On one of the dissatisfying occurrences, there was clear evidence that the carers delayed covering a malodorous gammy wound and responding to us because after peeling off their simple band-aid, a fly flew away from its mucky nest, leaving its dirty babies behind.

On another occasion, I came into a resident's room to see a man, recently discharged from hospital with urinary retention. He stood up from his seat with his hands on his hips, wearing only his white fronts and a vest top. He had no care in the world thanks to his advanced dementia, yet I was concerned that his indwelling catheter was dangling down from the penis with the attached urine bag dragging on the floor. And yes, the urine bag was weighty and approximately 300 millilitres full. In the defence of the care staff, they haven't had a catheter user in their residential home for a long time. I had to justify to the shift leader that the catheter must be hooked onto a retaining strap on the thigh and have the urine bag attached to the lower leg with two other straps. Neither the senior carer nor the non-English speaking staff members on shift could understand what was meant by my instructions initially, which was quite worrying because of the high risk of penile erosion developing. I'll let you look that up with the images displayed on good old Google.

There've also been some more disturbing instances I've heard from other healthcare workers learning about a foreigner being hired by a home without having a valid working visa, and this person left his 'job' after a few months and immigrated back to his own country before the police picked up on it. That reminds me of the care manager imposter of a local home I used to visit who was performing medical procedures on their residents while falsely claiming that they were still on the NMC register and on the way to becoming a doctor.

Regarding falsification, there have also been horror stories of paperwork being falsified. By that, I mean adequate food and fluid intake documented on malnourished residents, two hourly turns being ticked for residents with worsening bed sores, unexplained finger-mark bruises, and fall incidences not being recorded. As mentioned in NICE guidance in 2020 and in a section in my previous book, falls are something to take extremely seriously regarding risk assessment with our patients because fall-related injuries are said to be the main cause of fractures in the elderly. Falls can lead to deteriorated mobility, negatively impacting future independence and quality of life. In the latest statistics, when you get above 65 years of age, you're 30% more likely to have one fall as a minimum each year, and when you get above 80 years, the expectations are 50% for having at least one fall each year.

On the other hand, being a carer is an exceedingly thankless job, and in nearly all my visits to residential homes, I've had a pleasant experience with the hard-working care staff, who are few and far between. The above instances I've mentioned are a rarity, but unfortunately, they do still happen, and I'm highlighting them because they need to be safeguarded and brought to the attention of the Care Quality Commission (CQC) if known. Healthcare professionals must advocate for their patients' safety, who should always be treated with dignity and respect.

CHAPTER 18
REPORTING ABOUT THE PRESSURES

Monday, 6th February 2023

I took a colleague around with me on visits today. They overdid it at a family gathering yesterday evening and ended up having a hangover and were not fit to drive. The shift lead just thinks that their car needs fixing at the garage. We got through the double-up visits quicker, if nothing else.

Friday, 10th February 2023

Very occasionally, I hear stories of a patient groping a female nurse's bottom and giving saucy suggestions. It's never acceptable for either sex, particularly when patients have the mental capacity to be responsible for their actions. I'll always advise the nurse to safeguard this type of thing if it occurs. But regardless of the service user's capacity, it can psychologically impact the abused medical professional, potentially causing a downfall in their work and personal life.

Wednesday, 15th February 2023

Another responsibility I'm beginning to master as I advance as an Enhanced Wound Care Nurse is analysing and closing incident reports submitted by my team members about pressure ulcers. These reports are regarding either pressure ulcers seen on admission or (in the more concerning reports) pressure injuries that developed in our ongoing care with the patient. I get supported hours on a Wednesday afternoon each week to evaluate these incidents. There's become a prevalence of types of wounds within the community settings of our Trust, which haven't been well managed. They can lead to the consequences of hospital admission due to wound infection, sepsis and even fatalities. With each incident report I go through, I must check the timeline of care episodes by inspecting the progress notes submitted by each clinician. It allows us to see if we responded well to a pressure injury on admission or risk assessed the patient thoroughly and searched for ways to improve a patient's care. Not only to heal a pressure ulcer which developed under our service, but also to look for prevention of wound deterioration and avoidance of other pressure areas breaking down.

Suppose I determine that these pressure ulcers have led to a medium or a higher amount of harm to the patient due to the failings of our care. In this case, I need to discuss this further in a reflective forum with the members of the pressure ulcer panel, including the Clinical Services Manager, the Patient Safety Officer, and the head TVN. The forum enables us to fully understand why each pressure injury developed in the first instance. When identifying the learning outcomes in each occurrence, we can see what we can do differently in the future to optimise successful patient care and prevent skin breakdown. The forum supports staff in being proactive rather than reactive, reducing similar themes and trends, and getting the best learning possible from events and case studies. These discussions aren't all doom and gloom, though. It's designed to be a just and learning culture with no blame. We often recognise what fantastic work we can continue to embed into our everyday practice. From what I've seen when investigating pressure ulcers so far on admission, I've seen that the team visited the patient within 24 hours of being referred to our service with a care plan and wound assessment set up early on to prepare effective holistic care going forward.

In contrast, when I've analysed the reports of pressure ulcers that have worsened since admission, I've seen many significant gaps in our care. According to the progress notes, I've noticed that the team didn't order the most appropriate pressure-relieving equipment in good time, nor did they offer sufficient pressure-relieving advice to the patient or carers. I've seen that the team didn't promptly refer to the TVNs for guidance. I've also seen that the team didn't provide up-to-date risk assessments to determine the patient's likelihood of pressure ulceration or the patient's risk of malnutrition, nor did they upload regular photos of the wound to state whether it's improving, static or deteriorating.

As we love taking images for our clinical records, a photograph only tells half a story and won't explain why an injury was sustained in the first instance. There are normally obvious errors such as the ones listed above that cause a pressure ulcer, and we must execute a comprehensive individualised care plan on our software, which should support each patient's holistic needs, their wound care regime, and any helpful advice to educate the carers on the daily care in the future. If we meticulously evaluate the performance of our services, though, we'll discover the major reason why there have been alarming gaps in our care that cause such incident reports. It includes staff shortages and a lack of time for nurses to work to the best of their ability to correct what's gone wrong, make a positive difference in a patient's life, and avoid these negative patient experiences from happening again. Staff are being pushed to breaking point and overworked, leading to these little details being easily missed.

Monday, 20th February 2023

More devastation floods the news feeds today about a 6.4 magnitude earthquake that struck southern Turkey weeks after a deadly quake devastated the region. The mayor of Hatay, in south Turkey, has said people are trapped under rubble. This is in the same area where a 7.8-magnitude quake struck on Monday, 6th February, killing more than 44,000 people in Turkey and Syria, and recorded as the worst earthquake to hit Turkey since 1939.

As destruction hit the news, it picked up death figures in the hundreds and thousands, with many more critically injured. Buildings collapsed in a large area, and people were left underneath all the wreckage. There's footage of those alive praying for others to be saved from local people and those operating machinery trying to retrieve the missing. The Turkish military is fully mobilised in an effort to save as many as they can, with the US also sending military at the aid of the helpless earthquake victims. There's fear and panic, and small aftershocks keep coming, with lines of ambulances and rescue crews trying to help the worst affected areas where the walls of badly damaged buildings have collapsed.

I still haven't come to terms with Russia's invasion of Ukraine, one year on from the deaths of thousands of soldiers and Ukrainian civilians, while almost a quarter of the civilians have fled to become refugees in the UK and other neighbouring nations, with 90% of these being women and children. They can stay with people offering rooms in their homes through a voluntary *Homes for Ukraine* scheme for a safer way of living, allowing refugees to work and study with visas. Men between the ages of 18 and 60 cannot leave their invaded country by law, and many of these have joined the military to bolster their defence against Russia while the rest of their families hope to reunite with better days ahead. No-one knows how long this international conflict will last and what it may mean for the rest of the world.

Nonetheless, the recently horrific news makes me realise how thankful and blessed I am to live in a country that's currently free from natural disasters and not be faced with losing everything and relying on the shelter of a temporary mobile home or tent to survive. The increasing figures of these deaths also come as a sad reminder of the deaths from COVID-19 times and how countless more worldwide were living in terror during a global pandemic.

CHAPTER 19
THE IMPORTANCE OF ASSESSING PAIN

My service has been reviewing a 73-year-old gentleman, known by his middle name, Ronnie, and he has a tragic medical history of multiple strokes and a diagnosis of lung cancer and metastatic brain cancer a year ago. The gentleman has become too unsteady on his feet and has taken to his bed, especially since having a fall a couple of days before our first assessment with him. He was on the floor for 10 hours, and the wife he lives with suffers from dementia and doesn't know who to ring, so she waited for the carers to arrive. Through concerns raised to a social worker from our team and the patient's two sons, who live close by and actively support their parents, Ronnie is now set up with a care package. It comprises two carers visiting four times a day.

Tuesday, 7th February – Friday, 17th February 2023:

When our service did the initial visit for palliative support, the nurse checked that all pressure areas were intact. Still, they suspected a deep tissue pressure injury on Ronnie's littlest toe of the right foot, showing nothing more than black dots that were a couple of millimetres squared each. The nurse didn't need to apply a dressing and required the wife and the carers to monitor. At the same time, Ronnie denied any ongoing pains and wasn't taking regular analgesia apart from paracetamol at night. The nurse advised me to review as a follow-up, as the team's wound care expert.

As days went by, the wife and the care agency discussed the need for Ronnie to use a hoist and have his bed in the main living room as Ronnie felt isolated in his bedroom and found it distressing looking at four walls. Ronnie told the healthcare assistant who next visited how upset and depressed he was to stay in the bedroom 24/7. Moving the bed seemed tricky with the narrow spaces and corridors inside the small cottage, and the possibility was then considered of having Ronnie risk-assessed for hoisted transfers into his wheelchair, enabling him to have short spells of social interactions in a different environment each day. The healthcare assistant pinged a referral to occupational therapists to examine the safety of hoisted transfers. Whether or not Ronnie could maintain a relaxed posture in his side-lined wheelchair, he was grateful if this could happen.

Friday, 17th February – Friday, 24th February 2023:

When I inspected the toes of the right foot on the next visit, I noticed there were dark wounds on the tops of the third, fourth and fifth toes and a dark wound on the bottom of the fifth toe with mild bruising on the surrounding skin of the foot. The wounds were tiny circular scabs, which had somewhat opened before drying up, and I couldn't determine the base of the wound. Each wound measured approximately one centimetre squared, and based on the shape and appearance of them, I decided to document and report these wounds as unstageable pressure ulcers. With interaction from the wife, it was discussed that Ronnie had rubbed his toes against the wall beside his bed, and I could see markings on the wall resembling darkened wound exudate from the toes.

All wounds were dry enough not to warrant a dressing, and unless you're a pro at origami, toes are incredibly fiddly to apply dressings on. Touching Ronnie's toes has also become increasingly painful for him. As well as advising the carers and family to monitor these 'pressure' sores daily, it was also advised to apply ibuprofen gel to them every morning and evening as prescribed by the GP. There was already a pair of simplistic pressure-relieving foam boots in Ronnie's room, but they weren't being used. With Ronnie's consent, I placed on these boots, which primarily offloads pressure to the heels, but I was hoping they may also add some protection to the toes. After a few minutes, Ronnie wasn't comfortable because he preferred to cross his feet over. It then became apparent that Ronnie wouldn't tolerate a single boot on his damaged foot because his wife said he often wriggles in the bed to settle and pulls his socks off by his toes. This sparked more curiosity in me that not only was Ronnie being dishonest in my pain assessment, but there was also an undiscovered cause for the shooting pains from his darkened toes.

Ronnie's nutritional intake was reportedly poor, and low appetite was suspected to be due to his previous chemo and entering the palliative phase. He was looking emaciated in his red checkered pyjama bottoms, and a navy top, and I advised the wife to keep encouraging Ronnie to take sips of his chocolate milkshakes and a regular spoonful of his chocolate mousses but to not force this onto him as we're to promote comfort rather than cure. No concerns regarding the patient's bowels or waterworks were reported, but he's also now got anticipatory medications prescribed and stored at home in case he loses his swallow and needs any injections to manage troubling symptoms along the way. I also saw a Respect form stating that Ronnie isn't to be resuscitated in the event of a cardiac arrest and his wishes for future care to resume at home instead of the hospital or hospice.

As a further week went by, Ronnie became increasingly confused, and the palliative service assessed this as an effect of the brain metastases. Ronnie's wishes to be sitting out in the living room weren't going to be met because he was in no fit state to be positioned upright, and his cognitive ability was becoming too impaired to be aware of his surroundings and family members. I escalated a prescription request to the Equipment services to urgently authorise and deliver cot sides and bumpers on Ronnie's profiling bed; a suitable alternative to rubbing his toes against the wall beside the bed. It was also discussed in the recent handover with my nursing staff that there's a heightened risk of Ronnie falling out of his bed, and that's why his sympathetic wife is never too far away from him to monitor his every move, even lying on a settee opposite him overnight. The nursing team agreed that this new equipment would alleviate the possible risks of falling and the bumpers being particularly important to halt entrapment from the bed rails. I've seen and heard of accidents before where a patient with cognitive impairment got their head stuck in the bars of the bed rails in an attempt to climb and escape the bed. There've been very sad stories of this accident leading to suffocation and death, and we must prevent these incidences from happening again.

Friday, 24th February – Thursday, 9th March 2023:

When I next visited Ronnie's interdigital toes on the right foot, slightly open areas developed on the inner sections of the fourth and fifth toes, with a small amount of bloody exudate seen. I couldn't get confirmation from Ronnie anymore that he could feel the sensation of his toes, which I'd normally test with a monofilament pen, but I did notice how extremely sensitive he was to the wound care and kept flinching. I didn't detect any concerning signs of infection, but the surrounding skin appeared darker, especially at the bottom of the toes. The darkened areas haven't spread further up the toes, and I still suspected that the skin damage was caused by Ronnie subconsciously bashing his toes onto the wall before the cot sides and bumpers arrived. Ronnie was frequently moving his feet on the bed to get comfortable, and prescribed doses of liquid morphine are being carefully administered to combat the persistent spasm pains radiating from the foot. Ronnie's swallowing is deemed strong enough for liquids of syrupy or thicker consistency, and the carers and wife were advised to make sure the head tilt was applied on the bed during any episode of oral intake to avoid aspiration.

When feeding back these symptoms to the TVNs, deliberation about whether the dark areas on the toes related to vascular issues began to whirl around in my mind and prevented me from sleeping one night. That's why, in my next visit with Ronnie, I decided to check his arterial pulse sounds on his feet with the Doppler probe. The pedal and tibial arteries on the left foot showed faint, whooshing monophasic sounds and pulselessness in the right foot; unsettling readings from a peripheral circulatory viewpoint. The feet and lower limbs also felt cool to the touch and not normal body temperature, and there was a delay in the capillary refill of four seconds on the toes of the left foot when pressed and a longer delay on areas blanching on the right foot. The right foot's third, fourth and fifth toes appeared completely black today and felt solid like miniature clay sculptures. It was only on this visit that the wife brought to my attention that the toes on Ronnie's right foot were beginning to develop dark areas before Christmas when he could still sit out in his favourite armchair. If I had known this information sooner, I'd have arranged an investigation in the hospital into the skin cell and tissue decay of the toes. Based on the clinical judgment, I was sure that the toes were ischaemic and not damaged due to pressure. Ischemic ulcers result from an interruption of arterial blood supply to an area of the skin. They're typically painful, and unfortunately, even my very gentle touches of the affected toes seemed to cause sudden reactions of distress.

It was dawning on me that Ronnie hadn't been honest in terms of pain during his conscious state. A quote that struck a chord with me, which I first heard in a uni lecture, was from Margo McCaffery, a former member of the Oncology Nursing Society and a leader and pioneer in pain management for nursing. McCaffery stated that pain is where the patient says it is and occurs whenever the patient says it does. It made me realise that we must trust what our service users tell us.

However, what about situations where the patient can no longer speak out? In times before a patient is completely powerless and unaware of their feelings or surroundings, we can look out for signs of pain, which can be even more straightforward to identify to a skilled clinician, though they are easily undetected to others. These autonomic signs of pain can include frowning of the face, grimacing, wincing, eye tightening or closing and distorted facial expressions like furrowed brows, a nose wrinkling or the corner of a lip being pulled inward. Ronnie was ticking the boxes for some of these features. In terms of palliatively treating this medical condition at home under a short prognosis, it was agreed with the GP to treat the ongoing pain symptoms with a 24-hour infusion of morphine alongside anti-psychotic medication, operated on a syringe driver and to be titrated accordingly to maintain a sedative state; the kindest intention in Ronnie's best interests. The syringe driver started operating in the late afternoon. On the same day, I spoke to the family to pre-warn them about the probable complications that come with ischaemia of a body part. As well as pain symptoms, there may also be the complete loss of that body part.

These flimsy, black, withering toes kept me up at night and made me think: "Well, what if it just snaps and drops off? Do we just put it in our white waste bags and forget that it ever happened, and then that cytotoxic crud could be an environmental risk?" On my work laptop, it felt wrong to look up "how to dispose of a body part?" It would be considered very suspicious, and I'd probably get reported for having psychopathic behaviour. Instead, I referred to the Disposal of Healthcare Waste policy and went to the TVNs for guidance on the protocol for how we deal with anatomical waste, such as body parts that fall off.

I'm glad I gave the pre-warnings to the patient and their family because, on my next visit, the two smallest toes continued to shrivel up like thin sticks of charcoal. These toes snapped off in my gloved hand like a wafer biscuit, no matter how delicate I tried to remove the loosely applied dressings, and thankfully, due to the complete loss of blood supply to these former toes, there was no discomfort indicated. Ronnie appeared peaceful on his back with no more wriggling of his limbs and his eyes fully closed and completely nil by mouth, only to have his mouth regularly moistened with a toothbrush. My previous conversation with the TVNs was timed to perfection, and I brought with me a yellow clinical waste bag today, in which I placed the loose ischaemic toes; I double-knotted the bag and then put the bag in a sealed container with a red lid and with the large sticky label on the box it was identified to destroyed at high temperature for incineration only. I advised the wife to store the container somewhere safe in the house until the Waste Management service can collect it. The waste management team can only take collections on Fridays, and the family will have to live with the anatomical waste longer than they would've wanted.

The recent TVN advice also helped in an older case with Melissa, a patient whose left heel had turned entirely black and necrotic, induced by constantly digging their heels into firm wooden floorboards while glued to the TV during the daytimes. Just like Ronnie, they also had arterial problems, acknowledged later by the vascular consultant in the hospital when they started noticing developing ischaemia in their toes; they couldn't feel their heel at the same time, and the heel was significantly deteriorating from pressure damage.

The vascular consultant offered Melissa amputation, but she was stubborn and rejected surgery because she thought she'd have a better quality of life with all the dead tissues attached to her heel. When Melissa self-discharged and was referred to our service, she became a constant risk of osteomyelitis and sepsis in the subsequent weeks and months. To be fair to her, Melissa had already had a heart attack and required angioplasty the previous year and with the addition of congestive heart failure in her medical background, Melissa didn't believe she would've survived the surgery to her heel under general anaesthetic. In the care that followed, I wondered whether they regretted what they refused in the hospital before entering the palliative phase with the community nurses.

As a result of this lady's misfortune, they were left with a large necrotic plaque, which continued to lift until, eventually, it would drop off like a piece of crispy meat and gristle from a chicken drumstick, sliding off the bone. When the necrotic part of the heel was completely debrided away, it was later collected by the waste management service in a yellow clinical waste bag for incineration. This left the remaining part of the heel with a thick plug of boggy, gooey slough, resembling melted camembert in the thin, round, wooden containers it's typically served in. The smell remained malodorous. An ammonia-like stench of a spoiled blue stilton. And on that note, I'm sorry I'm describing rotten flesh and manky wounds as types of food. It happens to be the first thought of being a foodie, and I'm writing on an empty stomach.

Monday, 13th March 2023

One of Ronnie's sons contacted our service a couple of days later. It was news we were expecting and what all parties were gladdened by. Ronnie had passed away comfortably in his sleep. As always, in these situations, we offered our condolences and advised the family to call our office number again if they requested any support in their bereavement.

CHAPTER 20
WHEN AN INCIDENT BECOMES SERIOUS

Wednesday, 22nd March 2023

The Francis Inquiry report, published on February 6th 2013, examined the causes of the failings in care at Mid Staffordshire NHS Foundation Trust between 2005 and 2009. The report made 290 recommendations, including openness, transparency and candour throughout the healthcare system. It revealed the fundamental standards for medical providers and was designed to improve and guide compassionate and committed care with stronger leadership. The Francis report embedded more of a culture in healthcare where any suspicions of a service failing in the delivery of care for a patient are investigated. This is no different from the pressure ulcer forums in which I've had increased involvement.

There was a recent incident report regarding a pressure injury that developed and deteriorated under the care of the community nursing team and was suspected to have caused moderate harm to the patient or worse. This occurrence was scrutinised in a pressure ulcer panel hosted by the Clinical Services manager, my team's matron, a TVN and safeguarding leads. I was also in attendance as the team's reviewer of the case. The event was regarding Tony, a 78-year-old gentleman who was visited regularly for wound care on his coccyx, where the pressure damage occurred. Tony lacked the capacity to make any decisions due to his advanced Alzheimer's dementia. When the community nurses took over his care, all interventions had to meet the patient's best interests.

Tony also had a malignancy in his prostate and was to be treated palliatively under the GP's referral. Initially, the nursing service was planning weekly telephone calls to Tony's wife as an opportunity to evaluate him, which turned into monthly check-ups as Tony seemed stable at the time, at the beginning of January 2021, and was still attending the local day centre three times a week. This continued until the day centre stopped running in October of that year due to COVID. While this happened, Tony suffered a chest infection and spent much more time in bed with only brief spells in his armchair in the daytime. The nursing team kept Tony on routine palliative support calls, writing that all pressure areas on his body remained intact. By the end of 2021, the carers and the wife contacted the team occasionally, stating that Tony's bottom was getting red and sore-looking.

Palliative support calls continued, and information on good skincare and pressure relief was only said over the phone.

When it got to the spring of 2022, the wife raised concerns again that her husband's skin was vulnerable, and the redness wasn't going away, and she stated that a plaster was applied to the bottom. At this stage, there was still no planning for a nurse visit to determine if there was indeed a wound and whether a medical dressing would be appropriate. Nor was it explored who applied the plaster, and the triage nurse advised that the wife should continue with what they were doing, monitoring the skin and reporting any further anxieties if necessary.

A couple of weeks later, the wife was even more perturbed and insisted a nurse come out. Thankfully, a visit was planned on the same day. The practitioner reviewing Tony, lying on their double bed and foam mattress, had determined that there was just a scab, which was deemed "nothing much to worry about" with non-blanching redness to surrounding skin. After reiterating advice on skincare and pressure relief, Tony returned to fortnightly phone calls, even though a carer also noted that standing transfers from bed to chair were becoming difficult. Tony was only assigned a single carer, operating on her own, with Tony resting on a low-level double bed. From the outside looking in, Tony was seemingly weakened and dependent.

Several days later, a member from the care agency reported that the skin on Tony's sacrum was now open. A nurse visited on the same day, and a photo of the new wound wasn't taken for clinical documentation. The nurse described the wound as an unstageable pressure ulcer covered with tissue necrosis and a severe deterioration over a couple of weeks. Twice-weekly appointments were then planned, and an order was placed for an equipment services technician to replace a static foam mattress with an enhanced airflow mattress.

On the next visit, the healthcare professional who came to the house discovered Tony asleep in his chair. The wife denied wound care being provided at that time because she didn't want to disturb her husband with a hoisted transfer back onto the bed for treatment.

The following week, the wife again rejected Tony for wound care on the bed because he was asleep and didn't want the nurse troubling him. The team decided to safeguard the wife, and rightly so, in my opinion, because she was refusing important care for her husband for irrational reasons and not acting in the patient's best interests. The community nurses also agreed with the palliative nursing team to start to make a fast-track application for the Local Integrated Care Board to determine eligibility for a live-in carer to be at home 24/7 to offer respite to the wife who was at breaking point and to assist with safe patient handling on the bed alongside each carer who attends four times daily.

These two virtuous decisions demonstrated advocacy towards the patient, although in both visits where wound care was declined, the nurse didn't reschedule a visit the next day. Perhaps if this had been achieved, then measures could've been implemented sooner to prevent the wound getting bigger and worsening. When I saw this gentleman, my only review of him (because I'd just joined the team a couple of weeks before, during my induction), he was severely frail and completely bedfast. He had rapid weight loss and merely taking sips of fluid from a baby beaker assisted by his distressed wife or the carer, depending on who was in the room with Tony.

When the caregiver and I turned his cachexic body over, I was horrified at the gaping hole in the tailbone area. It was exposed without a protective covering of a dressing. There was also deep tissue damage to the mid spine and a category two pressure blister on the left heel. It instantly made me wonder how often body map checks were being done. In what periods is the carer turning the patient on the bed? The sacral wound was clearly at category four pressure damage and had brown staining in and around the wound bed from faecal contamination and small areas of pale bone exposure in the centre, which was firm on touch with my wound probe. The wound was malodorous on inspection, with angry lobster redness to the fragile surrounding skin. Each time I dabbed the cavity with gauze soaked in saline, Tony kept flinching in his feeble foetal position.

I dressed the wound with an antimicrobial of liquid medical honey syringed into the cavity with a fibre dressing to soak up any exudate. I applied a lollipop of liquid barrier film around the fragile surrounding skin, acting as a covering against any moisture damage. I then covered the wound site with an adhesive dressing containing an absorbent foam patch in the middle to avoid any leakage from the wound. I also forward planned daily visits for wound care and placed pressure-relieving boots on both his heels. I expressed to the carer the importance of repositioning Tony on the bed with specialised pillows and cushions, which are handy to assist with 30-degree tilts if this isn't being managed; all for pressure relief purposes for the whole body, however, these interventions were addressed too little, too late. All the physical observation readings were unsurprisingly all over the place, and Tony was at dangerous risk of sepsis from the wound critically colonised with bacteria and pathogens.

What's surprising was the inability to find a Respect form completed by the GP to consider whether Tony would remain comfortable at home or be escalated for emergency care. I left my concerns with a blue-light call for the paramedics to assess further and for the on-duty doctor at the local surgery to analyse what happens next in the care journey. When I checked Tony's clinical notes on an office desktop the next day, I could see that the admin staff had already notified that Tony was admitted to the hospital due to suspected pneumonia, which might explain why he sounded wheezy with low oxygen saturation levels, sweating in the bed with a high temperature. Three days later, Tony regrettably passed away in hospital.

In the pressure ulcer panel, all members, including myself, weren't convinced that pneumonia alone was the cause of Tony's death. They believed that a contributing factor was his horrible wound, showing clinical signs of infection. The panel wholeheartedly felt that the nursing service could've prevented a sad conclusion at an earlier stage in the timeline of care. Many learning outcomes emerged from the forum, which I needed to discuss with my colleagues in the next team meeting. This included the importance of taking regular photos to determine the wound description and when there were changes in appearance. They missed opportunities to respond with a visit under 24 hours when a family member was putting up barriers. The missed opportunities of reviewing pressure areas at an early stage when the patient is at a worrying risk for developing bed sores. Referring to the experts on tissue viability when the wound started revealing signs of deterioration and examining a patient's general well-being with physical observations was another piece of vital feedback for the team.

Were the caregivers aware of the severity of pressure ulcers and the consequences of the patient not complying with wound care and other nursing advice? All wounds are an infection risk, which has the possibility of poisoning the blood and causing symptoms of life-threatening sepsis. Discussing through the red flags for sepsis (fever, breathlessness, extreme shivering and muscle ache, new confusion, passing little to no urine in a day, pale or mottled skin and feeling like they might die) with the use of our Trust's awareness leaflet will enable a faster escalation of urgent medical attention for better survival rates of our patients, especially when nurses aren't available. If consent is gained, presenting photos of the nastiness of a wound to the patient or carers can be another good way of igniting a rocket up their backside to follow rather than ignoring useful nursing advice. A picture speaks a thousand words!

The events of Tony's care established the sheer magnitude of how crucial it is for a nursing team to be well-led and well-staffed. Communication is critical in achieving this, and team meetings and handovers are necessary to get to grips with all our patients on the caseload. Anyone we're concerned about must be spoken about. In my eyes, this case was highlighted as a *serious incident*. Wholly preventable, though in the current landscape of NHS services running with inadequate financial backing from the government, it's not surprising that serious incidences like this slip through the net in the nursing world.

CHAPTER 21
OPPORTUNITY TO SELF-REFLECT

Sunday, 9th April 2023

As my football season ends soon, hanging up my boots for my local Saturday afternoon side has been on my mind. This decision has been coming for a little while now as I haven't been getting as many minutes on the field for my local team this season, and instead, I've been watching players 10 or more years younger playing around me. I used to be the engine of a team, with all the stamina in centre midfield, playing 90 minutes consistently, but my body just doesn't work the way it used to. Maybe it's a sign of the times. Perhaps this is common when you hit the 30s. We're like machines at the end of the day. We don't run perfectly forever. And when you're working in a profession that is emotionally and physically demanding and kneeling on a hard floor doing leg ulcer care for over a dozen hours per week, it will take its toll on you much quicker.

Nonetheless, it's also soul-destroying when you can no longer be satisfied with a hobby you once loved. I've grown to hate my Saturday afternoons, and life's too short to stick with something you don't enjoy. I'll be keeping to my gym sessions and will go hobby-hunting elsewhere.

Wednesday, 12th April 2023

Peacocks were marching into the patient's driveway today. I nearly swiped my car door into one of their faces as I stepped out of my car and onto the patio. It would've been a complete accident as the peacocks so elegantly pose around with no care in the world. It turns out that the patient is a feeder, dropping their left-over dinner out of the window. No wonder there's a flock of them.

Sunday, 16th April 2023

Although I like the autonomous side of this nursing field, I can also feel lonely at times, and when I'm on a bit of a downer with life, I battle with my pessimistic thoughts between visits to the office and patient's homes. Long stretches of work without annual leave can affect mental health, too, leading to burnout – emotional and physical exhaustion – a barrier for all key workers giving the best care possible. I'm currently experiencing the effects of this. The compassionate care that I've provided has zapped my energy, and when I turn to alcohol at weekends, it

Opportunity to Self-reflect

occasionally brings out irritability and my frustrations to the surface. I can feel ashamed of my actions, recently falling out with a friend over something silly and storming out of a pub during the night only to apologise the next day. I don't want to keep repeating these events, which is also why I'm working more on myself.

Winston Churchill once said, "Success is not final. Failure is not fatal. It is the courage to continue that counts." I can assure anyone that sticking to a healthy habit of meditation most days has helped me to continue progressing forward in my job role. It's increased my focus and concentration at work, and I feel that I've performed better with a much busier caseload when I'd felt overwhelmed in previous years. The other benefits of having a moment of silence have been the ability to be more relaxed when under pressure and ready for a better night's sleep, which, in turn, will make you feel rejuvenated.

So, even though I've had a little setback this weekend, I have time today to self-reflect and encourage anyone else to spend time sitting and doing nothing with their life. Even if you just have two minutes spare. Doing nothing and simply sitting silently and meditating in this modern world is tough. It doesn't tie in with what we're often told: that more is better than less or that doing is better than being. Adding a moment of silence into a regular ritual will support one in becoming more rounded and in control.

Thursday, 27th April 2023

I've recently returned home from a lovely European holiday with a couple of mates visiting Bratislava and Vienna. We were sightseeing the impressive architecture, beautiful interiors, and artworks that the museums, castles, palaces, and cathedrals had to offer. I also indulged in the morning lattes, great food and plenty of beer tasting was had, too! It made me realise how much I needed all of this. To switch off work mode completely for a couple of weeks and focus more on my self-care. It made me understand that approaching the intense weeks of work mode again, I still need to find self-care opportunities. It's been fortunate that I've not been in the position to ask for time out and reach out to a support network. Instead, I usually work on my mental and physical well-being by spending time at the gym twice a week, and I also spend time meditating by using a helpful app on my phone.

If you feel like you need to work on your career development, then you could try shadowing other services, like I have, spending time with the vascular nurses and members of the diabetic foot clinic, who I refer to in my tissue viability role. Further back in the past I spent a day with the hospice nurses when I needed extra guidance in my delivery of palliative and end-of-life care. Spending time talking with the hospice nurses and seeing how they operated not only helped me provide the proper support to the patients in their last remaining days of need but also to the carers and families. It enabled me not to overload information for patients and their caregivers and to say it in a way that they can comprehend. Looking elsewhere gives you valuable experience of how other services function, and it also allows you to make contacts and forge relationships and opens you up to other career opportunities.

I've also found that having self-study time has really helped in my career progression, and speaking to your manager will enable this to be organised. They can also support you to attain the qualifications you need while continuing to network and do more research. Journals are useful for gaining knowledge and enabling you to stay abreast of contemporary issues in nursing. I've discovered this by signing up to the British Journal of Nursing, which supplies many interesting articles that you weren't aware of, such as closed incision negative pressure therapy for patients with caesarean section wounds and using a new-on-the-market dressing claiming to be the perfect dressing on hard-to-heal wounds based on clinical case studies.

Saturday, 6th May 2023

I still find that people cannot transition to calling King Charles "the king" and refer to him more as "the prince" under the former Queen Elizabeth II. But today, we came together in our households on this grey, rainy British day and responded to the words "God save King Charles," as his majesty sits proudly on the throne in his grandfather's crimson velvet robe, he took an oath, and shortly after, him and his wife Camilla, beside him were crowned King and Queen at Westminster Abbey.

Street parties in various neighbourhoods may have been a struggle under the bleak weather we're so often familiar with. Instead of that, mum did a lovely buffet spread in the daytime where we helped ourselves to many traditional nibbles, including sausage rolls, scotch eggs, a caramelised onion quiche, potato salad, green leafy salad, beetroot salad, coleslaw, crisps and cheese sticks, a cheese board of crackers, and homemade coronation chicken sandwiches in respect of the day. We also had a slice of Battenberg for dessert with some trifle on the side, allegedly one of King Charles's favourite sweets. Mum really went to town on the food, as she always does for big events. Later, my brother Chris and I went into one of the pubs in the town's market square and caught up with local friends, which rolled into the evening. We enjoyed the second of three bank holiday weekends for this month, which I'm sure those of us who aren't working them are greatly appreciative of this year.

CHAPTER 22
ANTICIPATING A TRAGEDY

Monday, 29th May 2023

For fungating wounds, the goal of the nursing wound care regime is palliation and not to heal the wound. It's about controlling the wound exudate, which is notoriously high in volume for significant wounds of this type, where up to one litre of fluid can be lost. It's also about controlling the pain that can be due to the pressure of a tumour against dressings or clothing or perhaps neuropathic pains radiating from a growing tumour or even the exudate oozing from the wounds may cause burning sensations to the surrounding skin.

Fungating wounds are generally very vascularised, and there's a chance that these wounds can develop a bleed through the dressings. And this risk is heightened for Colin, who had a large tumour enlarging out of the left side of his neck. Colin was aware of his tumour six months prior, which he explained started from garden pea size to a Brussels sprout size and now to more like a cauliflower size with its bulbous presence. This analogy comes from Colin's experience as a keen gardener and growing these vegetables in his allotment, with ownership now taken over by his friend and next of kin, Amanda. Colin struck me as a proud gentleman, always well-presented with a freshly ironed shirt, normally checkered, tucked into a pair of chinos or jeans and fastened up the waist level with his brown leather belt. No matter how much the tumour was expanding, Colin was making sure that this wouldn't tarnish his smart appearance, and he also wore a tartan neck scarf, ensuring that the extra thickness of the scarf was on his right side to hide the identity of the tumour for when he had visitors.

Prepping in advance for fungating tumours is fundamental, including checking that the vulnerable patient has DNA CPR ticked off on their Respect form. Colin agreed to this. He didn't think that the possible situation of being resuscitated after bleeding out was the morally right thing to do. The advanced care planning stage should also detail an escalation pathway if the wounds worsen. In anticipation of an active bleed for Colin, the nursing service made sure special medications were ready in the house. This will usually be in the form of adrenaline. A one-milligram in one-millilitre dose of this medication, prescribed in an ampoule, will be soaked in gauze and then applied with pressure to the affected area of a fungating wound for 10 minutes, which will activate the coagulation system and may decrease the bleed persisting. I needed to do this for Colin two weeks ago when Amanda called out the paramedics before I rushed to the house. I managed to stop the bleeding at the time with the addition of adrenaline, causing local vasoconstriction, and I resumed the wound care regime that the nurses followed. It involved the use of antimicrobial dressings applied directly to the open wounds, as well as charcoal dressings on the outside of the secondary absorbent dressing pads, which are effective in combating the malodour increase. The paramedics were grateful simply to watch my actions, as wound care wasn't their forte.

At this point, Colin had a tray of cat litter under his bed and downstairs in the corner of the living room. Our service gave him this advice as a good way of absorbing an unwanted odour. Colin also used a room diffuser and sometimes essential oils under our guidance, maintaining a pleasant smell in the home. He didn't want to over-use his deodorant, aftershave or washing detergent as an alternative in case it would cause any psychological impact on Amanda, who's often at home as his caregiver. She was warned that a perfume may trigger unwanted emotions after a loved one's death. Colin's been conscious of his shortened life expectancy when his oncology doctor was brutally honest that he'd have about six to 12-months to live.

There can be a mixture of psychological issues, many of which Colin had undoubtedly endured over the six months. There was a form of denial that something wrong was happening to his body in the initial stage, with a need to resume normal activities regardless of knowing the harsh realities of a progressive, life-limiting condition. There can be elements of fear of the unknown and what we or the palliative care service may have told him.

With that said, keeping things light-hearted and having a laugh can be important for the service user, their family, carers and friends under such circumstances. It can help the patient's loved ones recapture a fonder experience rather than a sad, heart-rending one.

Amanda kept saying how much of a strong, likeable character Colin was, which shone through in our visits with him, and he never seemed to be withdrawn from society and the dynamics within the home. Even though he never had a wife, husband or kids, and his parents and other relatives were deceased, he still had many friends in the village, including Amanda.

He was also never far away from providing humour, and I remember him joking, "Isn't it fortunate that I'm not an owner of a cat that may poop in the litter trays and add to this offensive smell."

On a Friday a month ago, I also remember him being upbeat and looking forward to the weekend ahead, and he said, "There's life in the old dog yet, George. I'm inviting some friends over Saturday night for a Chinese while we watch Eurovision, and you never know, I might join them for a G and T and a dance."

Anticipating a Tragedy

Since the episode of treating that small bleed to his tumour site with adrenaline, there was no *rebound* bleed once the effects wore off, and the medication wasn't needed in the several visits that followed. On a recent assessment by the GP, they decided to continue Colin on blood thinning medication when they considered Colin's past history of a stroke and heart attack and said that the likelihood of clots outweighed issues caused by a bleed. My nursing team had growing concerns that the wound had the potential risk of a catastrophic bleed. I had a long discussion with Colin and Amanda about the situation and that in the event of a catastrophic bleed to the neck, there are dark-coloured towels available. It's a useful idea to use dark towels to make the bleeding seem less dramatic. Otherwise, it would look like a murder scene and be even more upsetting for all involved.

I also advised Amanda that she'd need to contact 999 to escalate for paramedics to administer the buccal midazolam to help Colin remain calm and avoid any suffering through shock during a massive, terminal bleed. Buccal Midazolam was prescribed in pre-filled syringes for a time of crisis and only if Colin was showing signs of distress during an event due to experiencing features of hypovolaemic shock, such as agitation, hyperventilation, rapid heartbeat, or feeling weak or tired. Amanda said she wouldn't be comfortable administering this oral medication herself if she was alone with Colin and no healthcare professional present.

In unfortunate cases, outside of a nurse's visiting times, a terminal bleed from a fungating tumour has started, leading to a patient becoming unconscious within minutes. Patients can die very quickly before the sedation has started working. Colin's story sadly ended this way as the triage nurse learned from an emotional phone call with Amanda. She said that once she saw that the dressings were getting red and were sodden and started dripping with blood, she used dark-coloured towels to wrap around the side of the neck and pressed the wound, applying compression to stem the bleeding. Amanda reassured Colin as best as she could, cradling him while he was trembling in his chair. The reality was that Colin lost total consciousness within a minute, but what felt much longer for Amanda at the time. Amanda added that she called for an ambulance because she felt overwhelmed and didn't know what else to do. Colin was pronounced dead on the arrival of the paramedics.

Amanda managed to build Colin a rockery in the garden beside his pond. It was to be Colin's next project before he was diagnosed with his life-limiting condition. Amanda knew this, and she took comfort in sitting with Colin on the bench on the garden patio a week before his passing. Colin could see Amanda's wonderful work while sipping on a gin and tonic and smiling when a ray of sunlight was beaming down on them.

CHAPTER 23
THE FIRE RISK

Thursday, 1st June 2023

Finally, the satisfying news that more than one million NHS workers had been wanting to hear for a long time has come today. The Agenda for Change contract has been agreed upon between the nursing unions, the government, and the Department of Health and Social Care regarding nurses, paramedics and 999 call handlers. UK staff in these positions within the NHS will receive a pay rise of five per cent, backdated to April of this year. In addition, they'll receive a *one-off* NHS back-log bonus, and for the average nurse in band five pay, this equates to an extra £1,350; therefore, all our payslips will look superb at the end of the month. This non-consolidated award of two per cent of an individual's salary for 2022 to 2023 recognises the sustained pressure facing the NHS after the pandemic and the extraordinary effort staff have made to meet the Prime Minister's promise to cut waiting lists.

The agreement on the Agenda for Change contract comes at a time when the RCN had just recently sent a further ballot paper through my door, asking me to vote on whether to strike over the fact that the government and the Department of Health and Social Care hadn't come to agreement on a pay deal for nurses that was acceptable. Until now, every nurse nationwide has been belittled for all our hard work. There's been such a lack of respect for the NHS, the precious organisation run largely by nurses. My feelings alone had prepared me to participate in strike action again, but there were also some instrumental points in the latter part of the RCN's latest letter that made me certain to mark my vote with an X on the ballot sheet. This included the fact that there are record levels of nursing vacancies in the NHS in England, the inflation rates don't seem to be falling as the government claimed they would, and more than eight in 10 members reported not having enough staff at work to meet patient needs. You've only got to see the office at my workplace in the mornings with agency nurses ready to be allocated the many unallocated visits on the daily planners across all six teams in our region.

Tuesday, 20th June 2023

My vocabulary in my head or when I'm in the car on my own during work hours can be unpleasant, and without wording it on paper, it would sound very much like someone with Tourette's who's fixated on the F-bomb. Today was no different when I received the disappointing news that the developers of the new-build apartment I was moving into were way behind schedule and wouldn't have it completed until next year. Just when my shared ownership mortgage had been settled, and I was being billed considerably by the solicitors. I'm just glad that so far in my nursing career, I've not let swearwords slip out in a work environment with people around. Then, when the phone rings, I can quickly switch to a cheery voice and enter the office or the next home address with my smile back, meaning they'll never know how stressed, upset, or angry I've been.

Thursday, 22nd June 2023

The Bank of England's base interest rate is now its highest in 15 years at five per cent. It's a sign of the times. The last time we were hit this hard was when we went into a recession in 2008. Good old Brexit and the international events of the coronavirus pandemic and Russia's invasion of Ukraine have caused disruptions in so many ways. I feel it has contributed significantly to the high inflation the UK is experiencing and has attributed to supply issues. For example, due to shortages, there's upward pressure on energy prices and the cost of foods, such as grain and vegetables. Trades for building materials is an added example, causing housing not to get built in time and why the developers of the two-bedroomed apartment on a shared ownership property frustratingly fell through for me.

Shortages in medical supplies are another thing I'm frequently noticing when looking at the store cupboard. One week, we're low on sterile dressing packs. A different week, we're short on tape and adhesive foam dressings. Most weeks now, we're desperate for woolly bandage, a product often needed before the application of compression bandaging, and this is slowing down the healing rate of our patients with leaky leg ulcers and another factor in preventing us nurses from working at our full potential.

Wednesday, 5th July 2023

Today marks the 75th birthday of the NHS. This organisation might be recognised by many as "a precious institution" and a "national treasure," but I and plenty of other nurses fear for the future of the NHS and worry that it may not reach its 100th birthday. With the ageing population, numerous disappointed people on waiting lists for treatment and much of its staff unhappy with their salaries, we have good reason to assume the worst. But at this moment in time, it's still worth celebrating this milestone for its people.

Thursday, 17th August 2023

I've just started my four-day weekend, but I feel rubbish, sneezing and coughing regularly with a stuffy nose, and my body is starting to ache in places, including my head. So, I decided to do a lateral flow test. Something I haven't done for several months, and lo and behold, I get the two lines to show that I'm positive for COVID-19. Granted, I did see a patient yesterday who had also been infected by COVID for a whole week, but I thought I defended myself well against her and the husband by applying PPE with my specialised fit-tested mask before entering because I was warned in the triage notes. I visited them last to stop any spread to colleagues or other vulnerable patients and threw the uniform straight in the washing machine when I got home before showering.

That said, I dread that my second case of COVID isn't a brand-new diagnosis because I was starting to turn poorly earlier in the week, but I was putting it down to the common cold. I tested Mum as well this morning, and she's also positive, so my household is well and truly diseased by the invisible enemy. What's more worrying is that I went to a popular music festival last weekend, and the friend I went with also said they felt unwell today with similar symptoms to me, so that it could've been subtly spreading back then. I've now read news stories with scientists claiming that a new

COVID strain, known as the "Eris" variant, has begun, and we should all go back to wearing masks again. I really hope we don't get another vicious resurgence of the virus. For now, I'm nursing myself mainly in my bedroom and testing myself daily until I get a negative reading. I'll keep track of the dates written on the testing devices that'll temporarily live on my dressing cupboard in my bedroom, where you'll also see three pairs of scissors and a handful of used lancets that need to go into my sharps bin in the boot of the car. I can also see twelve pens and five measuring tapes that I've accumulated from reps of medical companies who've visited our office. Not forgetting the three rolls of tape. You're not a nurse if you don't have these things in your room.

Nevertheless, COVID has reminded me that it's still alive. It's never gone away since we first heard about it, and it continues killing and damaging people's lives through persistent fatigue and brain fog known as long-COVID. After a few months of not wearing a mask on visits, I'll make it compulsory to wear one each visit again because I don't want to take any chances, and I still want to protect myself as best as possible during my clinical duties. Where we've seen the virus intensify in the colder months, we'll all need to go into the winter with our blinkers on to avoid the NHS hitting a crisis with extreme pressures once again.

Monday, 21st August 2023

Doctors and nurses are accountable for what they do in the NHS trusts they work for and have the regulatory bodies they must answer to. Accidental mistakes can easily happen in our jobs due to human error. As clinicians, we must be prepared for the unexpected and have our wits about us. We must advocate for our patients' health and well-being; thus, if harm is purposely done to them, we must explore who the perpetrator might be. This might not necessarily be the friends or family or caregivers who are always around and who you expect did the harm. It could be a staff member in your service. We've only got to remind ourselves of the serial killers who committed such heinous crimes during their times as medical professionals, such as the doctor Harold Shipman and the baby-killing nurse Beverley Allitt, and now Lucy Letby will be joining Beverley's infamous title with life imprisonment.

If I suspect a staff member commits wrongdoings, I'll be whistleblowing by reporting the criminal offence and regulatory breach internally through my employer. For example, contacting the NMC, named as a prescribed person in law, or the NHS whistleblowing helpline number. Reporting can also be achieved externally via CQC, and concerns can be raised anonymously to protect confidentiality. These actions can save lives.

Friday, 25th August 2023

There have been over 50 fatal fire incidents reported by fire and rescue services in England since 2010 in which emollients were used by the victims or were present at fire premises. In most situations, the victims were over 60 years old, with impaired mobility, actively smoking, or bedbound. Using an air-flow mattress or cushion was a contributing factor in a few of these cases.

One story that struck a chord happened at the beginning of this month to Kabir, a 77-year-old retired manager of an Indian restaurant. He lived alone in a two-bedroom ground-floor flat and had a fire alarm system linked to a CarePhone facility (monitored 24 hours a day). Kabir was a regular, 'safe' smoker, using an ashtray to put out cigarettes. He had a longstanding psoriasis skin condition, requiring daily applications of emollient containing 11% paraffin to treat it. He had numerous visits daily from his care workers, his beloved daughters and the district nurses who had recently treated an ulcer on the left lower leg. Kabir wore a waterproof protector for his leg dressing when having showers, and he habitually used his dressing gown to pat dry his skin afterwards as it was softer than towels.

The alarm system was activated on Tuesday, 1st August, at 10:10 a.m. When the fire service attended the property, Kabir's daughters were expectedly emotional (with the paramedics) after being alerted by the CarePhone system. When the attending fire and rescue service crew entered the property, black, acrid smoke came from the bathroom. Sadly, Kabir was found showing no signs of life. With the Hampshire and Isle fire investigation team and input from the family members, the suspected fatality materialised the following way: Kabir was wearing his dressing gown that morning, and he went to light a cigarette after breakfast, but in doing so, the lit match fell and caught his dressing gown which set alight rapidly. Kabir got out of his chair in the lounge and went to the bathroom to find water to douse the flames. Even though his journey from the living room to the bathroom probably took seconds, his dressing gown was well alight, and it was alleged that Kabir struggled to undo it because the remains of the gown showed the belt was still double-knotted. Kabir managed to get into the bath, where he was found and showered to put out the remaining flames, although, by this time, there was little left of his dressing gown. One of the daughters alerted the ambulance, but Kabir was pronounced dead on the paramedics' arrival, having suffered burns on 75% of the body. The coroner's verdict was an accidental death, and the emollients had contributed to the speed and intensity of the fire.

The Medicines Healthcare Products Regulatory Agency reviewed new data with expert advice from the Commission on Human Medicines and found that there's a general lack of awareness of these fire risks despite previous alerts (with warning labels on emollients, especially products containing more than 50% paraffin) and evidence of misunderstanding the mechanism of risk.

Our service has now urged everyone to start using a poster that arrived in the office in multiple copies today, promoting to patients that clothing, bedding, dressings and bandages with skin cream dried on them can catch fire easily, causing severe and fatal burns. Emollients are available as cream, ointment, lotion, gel, spray, bath oil or soap substitute. They manage dry skin conditions such as eczema, psoriasis and ichthyosis. The poster advises that emollients are continued as directed, but raising alertness of the potential danger and how to keep yourself safe when using these products is just as significant. Staying away from naked flames and other heat sources such as gas, halogen, electric bar or open fires whilst wearing clothing or dressings that have been in contact with emollient-treated skin is the fundamental information from this. Those who smoke and cook need to be extra vigilant and ensure the emollient doesn't dry onto cushions, soft furnishings, and bedding, and washing bedding and clothing frequently at the highest temperature recommended by the manufacturers is crucial in preventing scenarios like Kabir's horrific story.

CHAPTER 24
ONE MAN AND HIS DOG

Tuesday, 5th September 2023

They say in our job that every day's a school day, and sometimes it can be through what you overhear in the office. Today, a healthcare assistant talked about a psychological way of removing warts using an organic object that'll rot, such as a rash of bacon or banana skin. This had been tried and tested for a wart on her son's finger, which surprisingly worked. In this case, a banana skin was used, rubbed all over the finger affected by the wart, and then buried in the garden. Each day from then on, her son was told to walk to where the banana skin was and acknowledge that it was buried, and they thanked it for working. As the banana skin rotted, the wart gradually disappeared.

A wart can last ages until it vanishes as the body adapts and finds white blood cells to fight it. Much scientific evidence suggests that psychologically, you can get rid of them by tricking the mind and encouraging the white cells, which the healthcare assistant taught her son to do. The wart virus needs a psychological smack in the face to get the white cells working.

Monday, 11th September 2023

I used to believe that once an acute surgical wound had healed, that was the end of the treatment journey for the patient; however, the scarring can have an emotional impact, and everyone reacts differently, which is important to acknowledge as a healthcare professional. Every scar tells a story. A scar might make someone feel scared and be a constant reminder of something tragic that happened to them. It can make someone self-conscious about how the scar looks on their body, especially if it's affected relationships that they've had. It may even make a person feel proud to have gotten through their surgery.

So, when I saw a gentleman with an above-knee amputation earlier and when I was getting them to observe their beautifully healed scar and to touch the scar, it was useful in promoting desensitisation and helping make the shortened limb feel a part of their body. Other people may have hypersensitivity to their scars, and if that's the case, they may want to use something else to touch their scar, but you need to be sensible in what you advise. For instance, a makeup brush could be gentle enough. Anything sharp and pointy, like a screwdriver, isn't so clever and can lead to another trip to see the surgeon. A speaker at a wound care conference taught the audience about the benefits of scar therapy, which can be in the form of massage techniques, such as using circular motions with your fingers around the scar and using a moisturiser in the massaging process. I've been told by a reliable colleague that Vaseline works just as well as the posher stuff like Bio-oil, and increasing your fluid intake will keep skin hydrated, too. We don't mean plenty more coffee or alcoholic beverages when we say that, either! It usually takes two years for scar maturity to develop. During that time, this advice I've mentioned will enhance the modelling of nerve regeneration and create vasodilation to increase blood supply to the area of concern. Giving the scarring more chance to smooth out and blend in with the rest of your healthy, intact skin and eventually becoming less visible.

Friday, 29th September 2023

Our kind-hearted diabetic gentleman sadly passed away six weeks ago. Even though his last blood results were a bit all over the place, the suspected cause of the death was cardiac arrest. Jimmy was already known to the heart failure service; he'd been experiencing a worsening in his shortness of breath, and the fluid build-up was increasing in his chest and his legs, although he kept leg ulceration at bay with the use of his compression stockings and leg elevation in his recliner chair. He had a dog named Daisy, an elderly border collie of 15 years old, and she was always slumped in the corner under a table and lying on her right side, with her face constantly looking in our direction with her glazed eyes. She watches attentively like she did in her glory years of herding the sheep together for Jimmy on his farmland. Jimmy praised Daisy for her patience and discipline on the farm and for making his transition into retirement more pleasant to manage when it was a livelihood he found so difficult to give up, though he knew he had to for health reasons. The nephew said that Daisy's been going downhill at a similar rate to Jimmy's health decline, and she's developed glaucoma in her right eye, has arthritic legs, and unfortunately, cannot always make it to the garden to do her business. One of the nurses saw this first-hand, noticing Daisy slowly and inelegantly carrying her tired self into the garden and taking a bit of a stumble in the process with her left hind leg giving way. The nurse said it was heartbreaking. Jimmy has intentionally been living in the closest room to the garden, the coldest area within the red-brick cottage, renovated from what was once a garage, yet it was the shortest distance for Daisy to walk outside.

When Jimmy was organising his advanced care planning, with the completion of his Respect form, in his care after death arrangements, it was decided that Daisy would need to be put down if still alive due to a diminished quality of life and no one to take care of her.

Jimmy has also decided to organise a woodland burial, to be buried in a biodegradable coffin, without needing rigid lines of plots or a fixed headstone. Daisy's ashes will also be scattered in the same spot. Jimmy's family have gained approval from the funeral directors, local council, and the environmental agency for this to go ahead at the local woodland, lying between the cottage and the farmland. It was a tranquil place which Jimmy relished on quieter days outside of farming, and he said how much Daisy enjoyed roaming there in her active years. Jimmy had never known a dog before Daisy being so enthusiastic walking through those woods in the mornings, in all seasons of the year; thus, it's only fitting that they're laid to rest together in their place of sanctuary. Another tremendously poignant story. The reason I know all this is because Jimmy's nephew invited members of the nursing service to attend the funeral since the coroners have finished their investigations and were satisfied that Jimmy died of natural causes.

CHAPTER 25
A LONE WORKING NIGHTMARE

Friday, 21st October 2023

I was asked to go out and visit a service user with necrotising fasciitis of their right leg, which required multiple skin graft treatments in the hospital. The severe diagnosis and treatment were a consequence of his recreational drug abuse. Their medical background includes heroin overdoses and alcohol intoxication and attending drug misuse clinics. As I've mentioned in previous end-of-life care episodes, there's a need for administering controlled drugs to help remove and avoid distressing symptoms. An obvious example is prescribing morphine sulphate to relieve breathlessness or uncontrolled pains, bearing in mind the patient needing them would need to be able to metabolise the medication based on their renal function and not have an opioid nativity. A patient in end-of-life care may also need midazolam, an antipsychotic drug used for symptoms of agitation. Suppose controlled drugs get into the wrong hands and are misused to induce feelings of euphoria. In this situation, it can be very difficult to remove oneself from an addiction so powerful and manifesting itself into a self-destructed life, as it has for Sally.

I arranged a double-up visit in advance, with a community sister accompanying me, and we had our security device turned on and attached to our lanyards due to the possible safeguarding risks associated with this person's medical history. A telephone call was attempted to Sally to try and make her mentally prepared for the visit, but there was no answer after a couple of attempts. When we arrived at the front door of the house, we were greeted by Sally's partner, Izaak, whose face was almost hidden in his bushy beard and the greyish brown matted hair flowing from his tatty woolly hat. When we walked upstairs and into the first-floor lounge area, Sally was sat on the settee, a lady with a gaunt, pale face and ginger straggly hair and who noticeably had a buck tooth missing when she spoke. Sally reported of feeling well but experiencing ongoing pains in her right leg.

When removing the dressings to the right leg, applied by the hospital staff, it was apparent that the referral wouldn't be a quick fix. At 49 years of age, Sally is left with life-long abnormalities, muscle weaknesses, and scarring from previous surgeries. It was the most deformed leg I'd ever seen, and it looked like she'd wrestled with an alligator. There were lumps and bumps from the knee to the ankle joint and crusted over cavities, still oozing thick yellow wound exudate. Surprisingly, there was only the faintest of odours present, but no doubt the tormented leg was at high risk of wound infections and cellulitis, especially when Izaak said that Sally picks away at her leg dressings now and again when she turns drowsy and bemused from all the "drugs" she's on.

Wound care consisted of a thorough bowl wash to remove all the crud that the leg was caked in, lingering on the surface of the skin, before plastering over our trusted honey dressings to all sloughy areas for antimicrobial covering. The leg was then covered from toes to mid-thigh with absorbent pads, woolly bandages, crepe bandages, and a lengthy tubular bandage to hold everything in place. Basically, 70% of what I had stored in my wound bag was used on Sally, and I needed to return to base after this visit to collect more supplies for the other patients I was allocated.

Sally's donor sites to both thighs, used for the skin graft surgery, remained dry and intact with slight redness, which was blanching and some evidence of scarring. Sally and Izaak were advised to monitor the skin, NOT to touch or remove the dressings, and to report any troubles to the community nurses via our provided service number.

The heels and ankle joints of both feet were inspected, and the skin was intact and blanching and Sally reported no other concerns regarding skin integrity. Sally's eating and drinking were said to be good, and Izaak discussed that she ate a cottage pie meal yesterday evening and toast with a cup of tea for breakfast. Physical observations were taken, including respiratory rate, blood pressure, heart rate, oxygen saturation and body temperature, and all her parameters were within the normal ranges. I also advised Sally to take paracetamol to take the edge off the leg pain.

The community sister and I stated clearly and concisely to Sally and Izaak at the beginning of the visit that the community nursing service follows strict criteria of only visiting housebound patients. When I initially asked Sally whether she could go outside and attend the practice clinic for further treatment, she said yes, but not at the moment because of her difficulty with mobilising independently and her ongoing spasm pains from the leg following hospital treatment. Izaak became very defensive when these questions were asked and explained that Sally would be too unsafe to go outside because of how poorly she's been, and he wouldn't want to be the one driving her to appointments.

In addition to these statements, Sally said that she returned home without all her medications after the latest hospital discharge, but she can still take her active medications, including amlodipine, to treat her hypertension because she had a stock of them at home anyway. Izaak then added that he wasn't pleased with how unsafe and premature the recent discharge was. He and Sally seemed keen to make a complaint against the hospital staff; however, at the latter stages of today's visit, it was discovered from reading previous clinical notes stored in a prescription bag that they were both lying to us. The discharge summary stated that Sally was discharged against hospital advice. Izaak supported this by saying that Sally found her way home by taxi. The discharge summary also stated allegations that Sally was taking cocaine and heroin whilst on the premises, but during this awkward conversation, Sally denied having any recreational drug use. Due to the evidence of Sally's ability to get into a vehicle safely, it was then discussed arranging a care car company to organise transport to the local practice. Both Sally and Izaak reluctantly agreed to this happening, and the community sister investigated this further on her return to the office.

As well as potential ongoing risks of self-abuse through recreational drugs, other safeguarding concerns were addressed today that I will raise in the next MDT meeting. Izaak said that apart from receiving financial benefits, they don't have any money, no care package at home and are relying on food banks to survive. The partner also said he is stressed looking after Sally at home. I contacted Adult services post-visit and reported to the coordinator a need to assess Sally's financial and care needs and the risks of self-harm and neglect. A social worker responded by saying that they'll review Sally on Monday. I also gave Izaak the number for the British Red Cross charity, which may be able to offer some voluntary support to them. The couple ended the visit being thankful for the nursing treatment and helpful advice they received, and I was relieved that there didn't appear to be any safety alerts on the surface to share with the team. The house contained a clean and tidy environment to operate in, with no apparent risks of needle stick injuries. It was evident that the couple had seen better days, though, matching with long, dishevelled bed-hair looks and teeth missing at the front of their mouths. There were holes in Sally's t-shirt and mucky stains on her tracksuit bottoms. These could all present as signs of abuse and neglect. Sticking to double-up visits with security devices in our possessions was still to be strictly followed, no matter how strained our service may be on visiting days. Doing this proved to be the correct decision.

Wednesday, 26th October 2023

Following my and the community sister's encounter on Friday, Sally required dressing changes on Saturday and Sunday because of the leakage from the multiple leg wounds. Over the weekend, it was reported from the two colleagues who visited that Izaak and his son were arguing quite violently. Although the nurses didn't escalate anything to the police or security service, they were on tenterhooks while treating Sally amongst the *effing and blinding* and death threats between the family members.

A Lone Working Nightmare

Then, on Monday, when two other colleagues visited, Sally was spaced out, with pupils like tiny pinpricks. She didn't even realise that the two nurses were treating her until halfway through the dressing change when she started juddering, and she snapped out of her zoned-out phase and suddenly muttered in her slurred speech: "Oh, hello! I didn't expect to be seeing you again today..." The nurses contacted the paramedics due to how vacant Sally generally appeared on the visit. Still, when the paramedics assessed, her physical parameters, including her neurological status, were stable enough for her to stay home after she came around with more consciousness. From this incident, we had increased suspicions that Sally was overusing her controlled drugs.

I was allocated to visit again today and doubled up with a community matron. When we entered, Izaak made us aware that his 25-year-old son was also in the house, who doesn't live with them, and Izaak said that he was taking drugs in the bathroom. Sally was calm on the visit, sitting on a dining chair in her bedroom, but she also had vacant spells, potentially experiencing the effects of recreational drugs. Izaak then said that Sally had taken all her pregabalin that she was prescribed, and she also took a large shot of green liquid methadone right in front of us before the dressing change proceeded.

I needed a bowl of warm water to wash Sally's right leg, but I needed to access the bathroom because the hot water tap wasn't working in the kitchen. This then created a full-blown argument between Izaak and his son, Dylan, with him urging his son to leave the bathroom and the house. It intensified and became a hostile environment with inappropriate language, making my colleague and I feel uncomfortable and unsafe. Izaak shouted that Dylan was under the influence of alcohol and drugs and was coming into his house uninvited for money. The situation escalated when Dylan abruptly burst out of the bathroom, and his maniacal, threatening behaviour got more ferocious. Dylan was shouting, "I will fuck you all up!" "I will fucking kill you!" He was also heard saying, "Get the district nurses to come and tell me to get out," when quarrelling with his father outside the room.

Dylan then came into the room where we were treating Sally, and there was a lot of shouting. Dylan pointed a sharp kitchen knife at the four of us ahead of him. He was as skinny as a rake with no clothing on his top half, displaying a skeleton physique, and the red elasticated trimming of his boxer shorts was showing above his black ripped jeans, which were drooped to the top of his thighs. With his squinty, restless eyes, Dylan demanded to have the Rizla cigarette papers on the windowsill at the other end of the room, yelling, "Just give me my fucking rizlas and I'll leave." He was fuming, sticking his teeth out like a snarling dog and again, the matron and I felt intimidated. We had no idea what this man was capable of, who may've had psychopathic tendencies.

Dylan then remained outside the room once the cigarette papers were passed to him. As shocking as Dylan's actions were, my colleague and I didn't witness anything physical between him and Izaak, but it was easy to assume that there was grabbling between the two from the grunting and rumbling sounds we could hear. That's not what you expect from a father and son relationship. Izaak came back upstairs, miraculously with the knife in his hand, which he put back in the kitchen drawer. The woolly hat was missing off Izaak's head, whose face was flushed and with his hair even more scruffy. He seemed shaken up about what had just happened, but there were no reports or sightings of bruises, cuts or stab wounds.

Sally grew more alert, the louder things became in the house, and she wanted to call the police. The matron and I felt extremely threatened and scared while completing the wound care for Sally, following our duty of care. I pressed the SOS button of my lone worker device as Dylan was still in the property downstairs, and we told Sally what we were doing softly to avoid Dylan hearing us, then told the security department to hold the line until it was safe to talk. I alleviated some of my anxieties with deep, controlled breaths and played a calm mantra in my head.

The son eventually left the property. The police were successfully signalled towards our GPS tracker when conversations with the security department commenced, consisting of questions requiring one-word answers.

I couldn't help but think that the partner instigated a problematic situation for all of us. He didn't have to go banging on the bathroom door demanding to get warm water. He didn't allow me to say I could use my saline pods as an alternative, which I used anyway. I felt he was making more of a scene because we were there. Izaak said at the end of the visit that he felt overcome with stress and that he didn't want to be living with Sally anymore, nor did he want to see his son, AKA "it" anymore, and couldn't cope with Dylan breaking into the house whenever he pleased, and getting money from Sally to feed his addiction. He wanted an escape route and added that if these outbursts continued, we would see a dead body lying on the floor on a future visit.

With Izaak revealing all of this, it really hit home about how serious these safeguarding concerns can become if they're ignored and brushed under the carpet. He said repeatedly in hysterics that he couldn't continue doing this anymore and felt everyone was at risk of harm. During Izaak's emotional cry for help, I could see Dylan waiting outside the front door for several minutes through a crack in the curtain. He moved on past the next block of houses shortly after this.

The matron and I gave stern words to Sally and Izaak, saying that in the present circumstances, our service cannot carry on visiting. Sally and Izaak claimed they weren't currently taking drugs; however, we found this unlikely with Sally's abnormally constricted pupils and

A Lone Working Nightmare

vagueness. Sally kept denying that she was getting illegal highs at home, and we halted any extra questioning on this topic as it felt like we touched a nerve with her, seemingly getting agitated with her responses. We also discontinued the subject of Sally attending the practice because Izaak became a little confrontational, even though we believed that was the best place for Sally to be treated. Thus, they can focus on her wound care needs without the social problems at home. When the matron and I left the property, we briskly rushed into our cars, leaving the road as quickly as possible while we were still in shock with adrenaline.

As we drove off the housing estate, we saw three police cars entering with their sirens on. When we returned to the office, we reported to our Trust's safeguarding team as well as Adult Services to urge for additional investigations because of the alarming risks of abuse between the patient, their partner and the partner's son within the current home, the high probability of self-abuse of the patient and the immediate risks of physical and verbal abuse directed towards nursing staff if our service were continuing to visit. The nursing service swiftly worked toward a plan to step away from caring for Sally so that she could be treated in a safer environment elsewhere. Our Clinical Services manager contacted Sally later in the afternoon to provide them with information on how to apply for care car transport, regardless of the financial implications, because if they can get their hands on recreational drugs and find the money to give to Dylan to feed his drug problems, then Sally can find the money to pay for the healthcare services that she needs.

No further contact has been made between my team and Sally. In the movie Patch Adams, the late, great actor Robin Williams said, "You treat a disease: you win, you lose. You treat a person; I guarantee you win – no matter the outcome," and in most of my episodes of care I'd agree with that. In Sally's case, though, maybe not. The road to recovery for Sally isn't going to be easy.

CHAPTER 26
THE FESTIVE PATIENT

Friday, 10th November 2023

Nurses can be the biggest hypocrites sometimes. I did a telephone consultation this afternoon to discuss a recent HbA1c result, identifying how a person's blood sugar levels have been over three months. I conversed with a particular patient that her readings were higher than they should be, and I offered the patient a referral to the diabetes prevention team. When I finished the call, I ate a Snickers and washed it down with a can of full-fat Coke. If I weren't clinging to a twice weekly use of my gym membership, it probably wouldn't be long until I was a Snickers away from crossing the type two diabetes threshold.

But then again, patients can be super hypocritical, too. Last week, a service user apparently couldn't attend their local clinic. When I rang the patient's mobile yesterday to arrange a house call (granted, on a different day than we'd previously planned), the patient said they were on the bus heading into town to go shopping. We've heard about these stories all too often before.

Wednesday, 22nd November 2023

Early on in my job, I realised I'd touch anything in homes as long as I wore gloves. Having a protective covering for where I sit and kneel should be followed, too. I often carry a grey circular pad to many houses to kneel on because the foam texture offers good protection and will prevent me from requiring knee surgeries and walking with a stick before my retirement.

The other thing with these circular pads is that they have a plastic case, which can be easily cleaned with a disinfectant wipe when I finish. I didn't have my circular pad today, and when I knelt on the ground and stood back up, my trousers looked like they'd been used to mop an entire house. I had wet patches on my knees, smelling of pee. I got out the alcohol wipes I had stored in the car and wiped the trousers down, and they're now on their second cycle through the washing machine. I won't forget my precious grey pad again when visiting an unhygienic home.

Tuesday, 5th December 2023

I went into one of the local care homes today to see a service user for routine wound care. On most of these occasions, I cannot help but notice another resident wandering down one of the corridors, wearing a dressing gown and slippers. He was reeking of urine and muttering to himself, seeming to think that the four walls around them hold a better conversation than any of the other residents or staff. As much as I was concerned that the quality of care could've been better for him, I pondered why individuals like this resident develop a nonsensical version of reality within themselves while blubbering gibberish. I know an obvious answer would be the degeneration of the brain over time. And then, I researched about the brain for my own peace of mind once I finished my shift.

Through my short exploration via the computer, I found that brain ageing and memory loss were once thought to occur because neurons died or stopped functioning. Neuroscientists believe we were born with a certain number of neurons, and as we get older, they reduce until permanently lost. The latest research reveals that the neurotransmitter dopamine can trigger the formation of new neurons in adult brains. These dopamine neurons move directly to the brain, are associated with higher brain function and could be the basis of mature wisdom. There's hope yet!

Between 20 and 90 years, the brain loses five to 10% of its weight, yet age isn't the only contributing factor to the shrinkage of the brain. It's our lifestyle that most certainly plays a huge part. According to the Framingham Offspring Cohort Study, chronic health conditions such as diabetes and bad habits – for example, smoking and drinking alcohol excessively – can accelerate brain shrinkage.

Other grim choices can trigger changes in the brain, too. A poor diet and limited exercise can lead to cardiovascular disease, reducing blood flow to the brain. In general, an unhealthy lifestyle may increase the chances of developing dementia.

So, how can we stay sharp as we age? A website I searched had identified six ways to help improve brain function.

1. Exercise your brain. Brain games, puzzles and brainteasers help create new associations between different parts of the brain, keeping it sharp. Other exercises that challenge the brain are using your non-dominant hand to do everyday activities, like combing your hair or brushing your teeth. It's not easy if you're like me and slightly cack-handed at the best of times.
2. Vary activities. Being physically active is tremendously important for brain health, but consider challenging your body – and brain – in various ways from time to time. Mix up exercise routines, and do something you haven't done in a while, whether that's hiking or joining a boxercise or spinning class.

3. Eat brain food. It's not easy coming up to Christmas, but we all know that a wholesome, clean diet will enhance all areas of our health, and there are many studies and an increasing amount of evidence that specific foods slow mental decline. Topping the list of brain-boosting foods is any food high in omega-3 fatty acids, linked to lowering the risk of dementia and improving focus and memory. And there was you, taking your fish oil just to keep your joints from hurting.
4. Try new things outside of the gym. Take up a language or an instrument, and memorise poetry. You could even take up writing like me! By asking your brain to do some new tricks, it keeps it active and ready to learn.
5. Volunteer. Research shows that this can decrease your stress levels and improve mental functioning. Volunteering enhances a person's overall health and well-being. This not only feels good, but it promotes brain health by raising self-esteem.
6. Socialise. We're social animals, and according to a recent study published in the Journal of Health and Social Behaviour, we need a mixture of ways to stimulate the brain, like social activity, to keep our minds sharp. This is particularly true later in life when ageing takes its toll on our memory and other complex neurological processes. The study

showed older, less sociable adults had cognitive and physical limitations compared to socially active people.

Tuesday, 12th December 2023

Occasionally, I quiz the patients about their physical observation readings. Just to add a bit of sparkle into their day. Some of them who become more regular with having their checks done tend to be almost on the money with their guesses. You get to know your body well as you age.

Wednesday, 20th December 2023

The nurses have been expressing themselves with their own medically-related Christmas decorations around the office spaces of our headquarters. There are mini snowmen made from rolls of woolly bandage. A mischievous elf with his hand covering his mouth and bent over a hole puncher with chocolate-coated raisins below to symbolise 'type one' bowel movement on the Bristol stool chart seen on the wall behind. There's an angel on top of the Christmas tree made from a face mask. On another wall space, there's a cardboard bedpan shaped like a reindeer face with inflated gloves used as antlers. There are also green and red tinsel lines in the form of the normal sinus rhythm that we would see on an ECG for someone with no heart-related issues. It's all still getting us in the festive spirit!

Friday, 22nd December 2023

We have a lovely patient who had 18 months of torment, starting with a tiny wound on the foot, which led to a nasty infection, gangrene, spreading erythema and ischaemia. This unfortunate circumstance led to toe amputations, foot amputation and finally, a below-knee amputation of the left leg due to the consequences of an infected diabetic foot ulcer. She hasn't let the misfortune get her down and has remained remarkably strong and positive throughout her treatment journey, with an admirably proactive and helpful husband by her side during the day. She's been getting into the Christmas spirit recently, and on the last few weekly visits, before we've treated her small ulcer of the right leg with compression therapy, she decorates her left stump with a knitted Christmas hat. On the first occasion, we heard of this through the visiting nurse who said there was a hat resembling an upside-down smiley snowman face wearing a stripey bobble hat. Last week, a green woolly hat was worn on the stump to resemble a Christmas tree with intermittent lights flashing and a thin strip of tinsel spiralling up. Today, her left stump greeted me with a brown beanie with two googly eyes, a red bobble in the middle for a nose and an antler headband. It was Rudolf, and with her consent, I sent a picture to my team's WhatsApp group for a festive morning greeting on the shift before most of us enjoy our Christmassy weekend with friends and family.

CHAPTER 27
THAT'S A WRAP

As I write this last passage of the memoir in early December, amongst the annual chaos of the winter pressures across the NHS, I'd like to wrap up with a multitude of noteworthy moments during the past three years of my nursing career. Some will be looked back on with a sigh of sorrowfulness or resentment. When switching off from our jobs, we then open our eyes and ears to the world's negative news stories, which have included the Russian attacks in Ukraine and, more recently, the battles between Israel and the Palestinian Islamist group Hamas, and these topics have prevented us from avoiding these unwanted feelings. Other times in these past three years can be reflected on with much pride and cheerfulness. I've highlighted in this memoir the positive contributions all the nurses have made within an organisation treasured by many, specifically those operating in fundamental community services.

In recent years, we've seen an upsurge of countless public servants demanding that the government offers them fairer, more reflective pay. We've seen the train services continue to go on strike and the Royal Mail's postmen and women, teachers and doctors at junior and senior positions. I believe the cost-of-living crisis and fuel and food poverty many have suffered have also profoundly impacted multiple strike actions.

Regardless of these challenging times, I can confirm that I've made another proud step in adulthood by getting on the property ladder, and I'll be picking up the keys to my new home at the start of the New Year. I realise how fortunate I've been to live under the roof of my parents to save up for this moment. Many nurses are in less fortunate positions, and we didn't need to be told about the crisis in the health service that we've lived through, especially when the rise in inflation was increasing in the UK. I commemorate the RCN for standing up for us, influencing the majority to go on strike to help end that crisis, and asking the government to fairly fund the healthcare sector and our profession, similar to what the other services in the public sector have been urging.

Thankfully, the government and the Department of Health and Social Care decided on a pay rise and lump-sum reward in June of this year, which satisfied our unions, and there doesn't appear to be any further disputes or strikes on the horizon. This is because the deal has finally shown respect and value to the entire nursing workforce who worked tirelessly throughout the global pandemic to assist in keeping everyone safe, and the government started to recognise that nursing staff have faced financial constraints in the cost-of-living crisis. They've realised the importance of preventing a continuation of dire consequences for our workforce regarding recruitment and retention and, in turn, patient safety. A lack of pay has no doubt affected the chances of nurses joining or staying in the NHS.

With that said, in a British Journal of Nursing article written in early 2023 by Jeanette Milne (Associate Director of Nursing Delivery of Northumbria Healthcare NHS Foundation Trust), she stated that there have been other factors. I agree with all the points she brought up because I've experienced them in my career. These points include staff shortages, a lack of recruitment, and poor team working conditions.

Despite this, whenever I'm summoned to help someone in the community, I follow the phrase, "Be the nurse you'd want as a patient." And we receive compliments in return for all the wonders we provide for our service users. Almost always, a meaningful "thank you" from them or their caregivers when we exit their door for the last time. The praise for the successful delivery of care is a testament to the team's unity and devotedness to the service, with exceptional communication, the cornerstone skill we use when delegating responsibilities to each other and discussing patients we've visited in afternoon handovers.

With such pressure on top of our hard work and dedication comes the realisation of staff reaching breaking point. I've felt my body giving me signs at parts of the year that I need to chill out more, with symptoms of drowsiness, irritability and brain fog creeping in with a racing heart, sometimes feeling its palpitations until you relax into a sleep. There'll be those in our service who bear the scars of moral injury and need the support of our other amazing colleagues in occupational health and mental wellbeing teams. As I've mentioned, I've relied on meditation apps on my phone to help alleviate any stress and anxiety in my life. This, as well as exercising and socialising, has been beneficial to me physically and psychologically, especially when times get hard. Staying focused is key in terms of productivity at work because, as Florence Nightingale had rightly stated, "How very little can be done under the spirit of fear."

I cannot deny that the last few years have been unbelievably tough, with the organisation still desperately needing every one of us. As well as getting through a global pandemic, we've been hit with some of the most brutal winters on record. You've only got to see it on TV, where it's been publicised in the busiest departments of general hospitals. Nursing isn't just seen as a fundamental profession in the UK. Even Barack Obama has once said, "America's nurses are the beating heart of our medical system." For those leaving school and pursuing a career and their *calling* in life, it must be difficult for them to consider having a career in the NHS.

The pressures embedded into NHS nursing professions can easily deflate the spirits of its staff, but if you ever feel like quitting, just remember why you started. It took you being resilient right from the start, right from when you began your first placements, and you were learning every medical abbreviation, drug and clinical procedure whilst caring for your first-ever patients and trying to impress every senior around you. Resilience is one of the most vital personal qualities of a nurse. It's about turning up to work again in spite of the new challenges you face along the way. It's about working the next shift after being shouted at by a patient or their caregiver when the service may have let them down in some way. It's about coming in the next day after being involved in an incident which has been traumatic for the patient and their family, and you've needed to be the emotionally strong individual to make the critical decisions and to be the shoulder to cry on when you felt like you needed some support too. Like all other skills and attributes, personal resilience takes time, experience, and patience.

In another British Journal of Nursing article I read this year, a newly qualified nurse, called Heather, said that her biggest challenge as a newly qualified nurse had been the need for more self-confidence.

This was served with a side of self-doubt and a generous sprinkling of imposter syndrome. Heather then explained that as she gained experience as a Critical Care Staff Nurse, having a sense of purpose was valuable, with the incredible feeling of seeing people recovering from critical illness and knowing that you helped them in the process spurred her on to maintain a nursing career. The sense of purpose can be life-changing for people, yet there are also times when your confidence may take a hard knock, and you go home from a shift feeling inadequate and that you could've done better. These times can be upsetting for people, and I must admit that I can be hard on myself if a mistake is made. We must also remember in these times, though, that we're only human. We're built to make the odd mistakes and to keep learning and developing. Even I'm still learning to forgive myself. I need to remember that no-one's perfect, and I need to show myself patience because we're all on a journey. We must cut ourselves slack and remember we've done our best in difficult situations. You shouldn't have to bottle up negative thoughts or feelings. The NHS encourages a positive culture where there's freedom to speak up, whether that's about personal battles, whistleblowing, a staff member not acting in the patient's best interests, possibly causing them harm or discussing the potential flaws in how a service is run, all voices need to be heard.

That's a Wrap

Amongst all the chaos, from a personal, organisational, and national standpoint, I also see glimmers of brilliance every day, with little acts of kindness. These moments can be seen from colleagues or caregivers caring for patients with passion, commitment, empathy and enthusiasm. And every so often, the patients inspire me with their inner strength and optimism, no matter what the ills of the world throw at them. Many have fascinating histories, from Second World War veterans to former athletes, teachers and medical professionals. For these reasons, I proudly wear my blue uniform, honoured to care for such inspirational people.

Moreover, nurses can be compared to an iceberg. At any one time during working hours, you're merely seeing about one-fifth of what they're doing. They're geniuses at multitasking, even if it doesn't always go to plan. If you've not taken bites of a Mars bar while driving between patients and trying to figure out why Google Maps has navigated you to the middle of a field, then you've probably never worked in community nursing. The same goes for people who've never been in the situation of frantically trying to write clinical notes while answering their work phone to colleagues, doctors or distressed patients. An outsider looking into this profession may only see a few responsibilities, one being that nurses are there to manage medications for their patients. Yes, nurses do that, but they can also provide comfort and compassion without a prescription.

I've also learnt in my time in healthcare that having time for laughter is crucial, and hopefully, by reading my memoirs, you've seen the humorous side of this profession. Time for hilarity can be spent with your patients, their families with your colleagues, or even better, all three simultaneously! There are a lot of serious matters in the world, and a lot of seriousness comes in our job, which considerably dominates our working hours each day and each week. But finding moments for light-heartedness and some laughter will relieve you and others of some pressure, even if it's just for a few seconds. It can make a massive difference, and as they say, if you don't laugh, you'll cry.

Working within the NHS and nursing in general is clearly not for everyone, and as I've demonstrated in this memoir, it takes someone to be emotionally strong and compassionate. You also have to say a lot to gross out a nurse because they have cast iron stomachs and aren't squeamish, especially when bodily discharges leave particular body parts unpredictably. You must expect the unexpected. From an organisational perspective, you must make yourself aware of the financial burdens on the NHS, including the growing costs of hard-to-heal wounds, which result in long-term morbidity for patients, negatively impacting their quality of life.

During my time in nursing, I've seen many outstanding staff members going out of the office door, never to return as they said their final farewells.

Occasionally, this is due to retirement. Sometimes, this is to move onto a different, progressive role in nursing. Other times, it can be for a new career change outside the NHS. One day, I'll also leave my nursing service and the NHS family. But just like everyone else who's departed before me, we'll leave a fire still burning bright, with the team carrying forward our torch of knowledge, wisdom and bedside manners. The skills and values we hold dearly through our healthcare careers will carry on through to an ever-changing workforce, one that's hard-working, dedicated and passionate.

If you feel like you can display the same qualities and prepare yourself for everything I've experienced in my memoirs, then you should give it a go and try community nursing, just like me! If you find yourself lacking a challenge and craving a change, why not give it a go for those reasons? Change doesn't happen on its own. It's all about adopting a proactive approach. If you desire to be something and see it, then you can be it. It all starts with belief, passion, and determination to get where you want to be in life, and even though I never imagined myself as a healthcare professional in school, my beliefs and values magnetically brought me to it.

Furthermore, the NHS and nursing allow for numerous avenues where you can progress your individualised careers. If you don't like one job you're in with the NHS, it doesn't mean you won't love the next job you apply for. Many opportunities are advertised, including my role as an Enhanced Wound Care Nurse, since the community teams have noticed a growing demand for tissue viability specialists. There's something for everyone, and you can develop a specific group of skills and knowledge to be a shining asset for your chosen workforce. That's the beauty of nursing!

ACKNOWLEDGEMENTS

To the wonderful integral care team operating in the community. From the management staff to the community matrons, the sisters, all the registered nurses, the associate practitioners, the healthcare assistants, the therapy staff, the clinic staff, and the administration teams. It's a pleasure to work with you all on a day-to-day basis. You're all amazing!

To the tissue viability nurses – the kings and queens of wound care – thank you for supporting me in my developed role. And thank you to the other Enhanced Wound Care Nurses who I've been able to bounce my knowledge and wisdom off with and to help prioritise the patients that take up much of our caseload.

To the agency nurses who have been a welcomed addition in helping manage the whole of the integrated care team's daily visits and prevent the service from getting too strained with burnt-out staff – thank you!

To all the GPs, the frailty teams, the pharmacists, and anyone else who works in the NHS and health and social care sector – thank you for the service you provide!

To the staff working in the administration department. You prove that multitasking to the extreme doesn't only apply to the nurses. Thank you for being able to listen to a lonely elderly person in one ear and complete email referrals simultaneously.

Working in nursing is a vocation, and whoever it is we care for, we have an essential part in their lives, keeping them safe and comfortable. When the alarm goes off on the morning of Monday's shift, you know it's a busy week ahead. You may, at times, have less than five hours of sleep in your system, and you're then deciding whether to make it to work or fake your death before you make your first step out of bed. Shifts are usually busy, and it's a little unsettling when you are asked to go out on those extra visits to see a patient with a new wound, and it turns out that their foot or leg is falling apart. The paperwork that follows can be just as horrifying.

I'm proud of my achievements as a medical professional and I'm thankful for all the support that has got me this far and how much I've learned, experienced, developed and achieved. But this is not just a shout-out to all the fantastic nurses and everyone connected with the NHS.

Acknowledgements

It's also an enormous shout-out to all other key workers who are significant in helping those who cannot help you back. Everyone working in health and social care has highly demanding and challenging jobs. As we should know by now, they are crucial jobs to many people and very rewarding.

For all the inspiring, welcoming, and kind-hearted patients and caregivers whom I've had the joy of working with. Thank you for allowing me to reflect on many pleasant experiences.

Even the patients who were sometimes cheeky, troublesome, and non-compliant, thank you for giving me and my team those extra challenges in our jobs. It's enabled me to develop more and more in my career journey and write up the many compelling stories in these nursing memoirs. It's always fulfilling to win you over with our advice and guidance, whether that's to lay off those sugary treats if you have diabetes. And to constantly ask you to elevate your swollen legs and take your diuretics even though you must risk rushing to the loo. And to encourage you to wear your compression hosiery, which does NOT feel too tight. They are firm and supportive!

I send my deepest condolences to the bereaved who have lost a loved one. Never forget the memories you shared, which will keep their presence going.

To Sabeeh ul Hassan, thank you for your fast, efficient service and for making an intriguing book cover design with an exquisite appearance to add to my collection. It would look marvellous on anyone's book self.

To the brilliant Sophie Hanks, thank you once again for your formatting skills and for creating the professional layout and structure of my work, from page to page, before my publication.

To Goldfinch Books, thank you for being such a welcoming bookstore in my hometown and a platform for giving me useful author-related advice and allowing me to use your bookshelves to promote my books, which has been an added boost in attracting the attention of readers alongside social media.

Thank you to everyone else who's supported me through my journey as a self-published author. That includes Jane and Sharon (the two incredible TVNs I work with) and one of my non-medical friends, Louisa. You were my star proof-readers, who helped give me feedback after a couple of rounds of editing, ensuring the book was on the right track with no errors in my medical language.

Most of us have thought of an idea overnight, which we believed was glorious at the time but turned out to be silly or regretful. Each of the self-published books I've written

Acknowledgements

contains many three a.m. ideas. People have asked me: Do you regret writing and self-publishing books? Was it all worth it? To answer those questions, I say, no, it wasn't regretful, and I'm glad I did it.

It's the feeling of personal achievement I've got out of being a self-published author and for persevering through many challenging experiences and coming out the other side with success. Each time I receive a great review from a happy reader of my books, it makes my day and all the effort worthwhile.

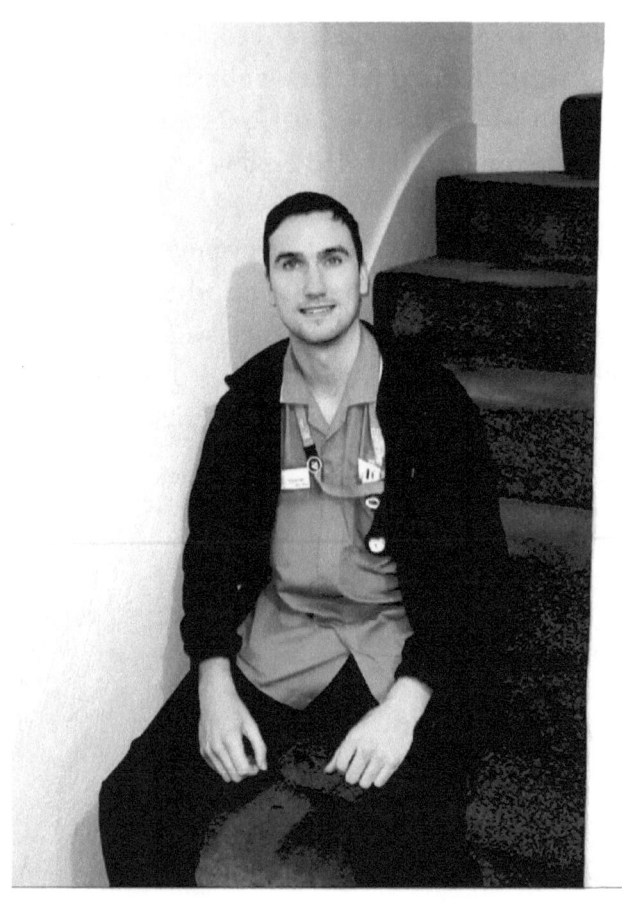

Picture taken at the end of 2023 after another busy year of being a community nurse.

AUTHOR BIO

George is the writer of three self-published books. His first book titled: *The Unplugged Summer* was an experimental piece, which gave a true account of himself at an earlier stage in his life. At the same time of self-publishing his first book, George accomplished his post-graduate degree 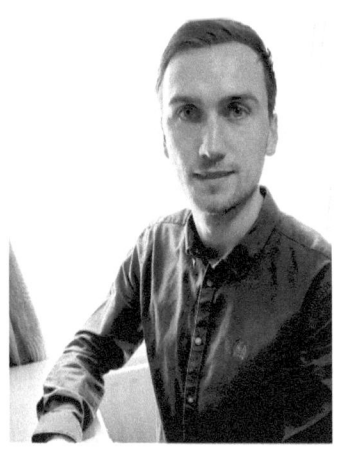 in nursing and graduated from the University of Southampton.

Throughout his first couple of years as a qualified nurse, George then wrote his second book: *Hidden Heroes of our Community*. This book provides multiple reflections of how the coronavirus outbreak altered his occupation as a healthcare professional in the community.

The third book, *Beyond the Eye of the Storm*, is a follow-on medical memoir from his previous book, filled with more experiences in his life as a community nurse in the aftermath of the recent global pandemic.

Now approaching almost five years of nursing experience, George aims to continue making a positive difference in people's lives as a valuable healthcare professional in the community.

George Horner: PGDipN (Soton); RGN. Community Staff Nurse

www.ingramcontent.com/pod-product-compliance
Lightning Source LLC
Chambersburg PA
CBHW021056080526
44587CB00010B/263